Get Fit

through GARDENING

Jeffrey P. Restuccio

Get Fit

through GARDENING

Advice, Tips, and Tools for

Better Health Featuring the

Unique Exercise Plan to

Save Your Back and Knees!

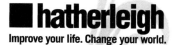

Improve your life. Change your world.

HATHERLEIGH PRESS is committed to preserving and protecting the natural resources of the Earth.

Environmentally responsible and sustainable practices are embraced within the company's mission statement.

Hatherleigh Press
5–22 46th Avenue, Suite 200
Long Island City, NY 11101
www.hatherleighpress.com

Library of Congress Cataloging-in-Publication Data is available.
ISBN 978-1-57826-268-7

Get Fit Through Gardening is available for bulk purchase, special promotions, and premiums. For information on reselling and special purchase opportunities, call 1–800–528–2550 and ask for the Special Sales Manager.

Interior design by Pauline Neuwirth, Neuwirth & Associates, Inc.
Cover design by Michael Fusco, michaelfuscodesign.com

10 9 8 7 6 5 4 3 2 1

Printed in the United States of America

This book is dedicated to all those who have helped me promote gardening as a lifelong fitness and wellness program since 1992. Thanks for helping me keep the dream alive.

—JEFF RESTUCCIO

Contents

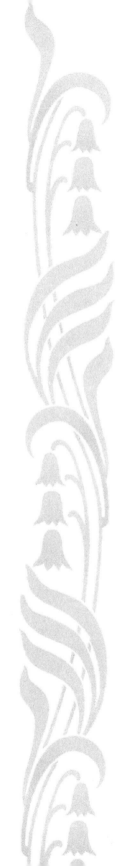

Acknowledgments

I WOULD LIKE to thank our two models, Robert Barton and Tanya Schafer, for their work in illustrating the different *Get Fit through Gardening* motions and techniques.

Get Fit

through GARDENING

Introduction

EVERY DIET AND fitness expert, including those selling you a "magic weight-loss pill" advocates "*changing your lifestyle.*" That's exactly what *Get Fit through Gardening* is: a lifestyle change. No other diet or exercise program can boast fresh fruits and vegetables as a result of your caloric expenditures. No other diet or exercise has a positive environmental impact from planting trees, composting waste, and recycling. No other diet or fitness program can create a more beautiful you as you create your own backyard oasis of stunning roses, mighty oaks, and delectable tomatoes, peppers and eggplant for your table.

I've been promoting gardening and fitness ever since my first book, *Fitness the Dynamic Gardening Way* was published in 1992. I've traveled throughout the United States, extolling the virtues of this funny-looking way of gardening. Yes, the exercise positions I promote such as the Lunge and Weed and the broad, legs-wide raking stance are unusual, and, at first, awkward for most people—but the techniques will lessen back pain and muscle soreness, reduce hand calluses, allow you to garden safely, and sculpt your body.

The majority of the more than fifty million overweight Americans would prefer a quick, simple pill or gadget that will answer all their weight-loss problems. If that is what you are looking for, then *Get Fit through Gardening* is not for you. I want you to embrace and accentuate the physical component of gardening. My fitness program acknowledges what 99% of other programs don't—this takes both time and effort. The *Get Fit through Gardening* workout makes time your friend. Success is measured in seasons, years, and decades, not days and weeks. It's your choice which aspects of this program you use. No matter if it's just the stretches and stances, the yard program, or the circuit-training program, you'll be growing something! With *Get Fit through Gardening* you can truly smell the roses as you become fit.

Get Fit through Gardening is not the way your parents or your grandparents gardened. By adding concepts and techniques from aerobics, the martial arts, resistance training, and other disciplines, I've created something totally new. You garden to exercise and exercise to garden.

The focus is now on *you*, not the plants. If you plant an apple tree and it dies two years later, that's okay. If you plant a bed of flowers and only 75% bloom, that's okay too. Your objective now is to use your garden as a tool to help you achieve the health benefits you've always wanted—without leaving the yard.

Gardening Isn't Good For You Unless You Do It Correctly

Most articles written on garden and exercise simply note that gardening is good exercise. When you garden, you sweat a lot, you're active, burn calories, and tone your muscles. That's all good—but for most people, bad habits and bad technique combine to cause back and muscle strain.

Most gardeners never stretch before they garden. They over-work the same muscles over and over with monotonous movements. They garden using primarily their arms and not their legs. They stoop over to pick up things. With the *Get Fit through Gardening* workout, traditional gardening is transformed into a lifelong fitness program. *Get Fit through Gardening* concepts are introduced, many borrowed from other disciplines such as aerobics, weight training, and the martial arts. Others have been developed from the form and techniques you already use while gardening.

Poorly designed tools are yet another roadblock to getting fit while gardening. Rakes, hoes, and cultivators, all with short handles under 57 inches, are the main reason gardeners stoop over and injure their lower back while gardening. Personally, I recommend a handle that's a full 72 inches. Using ergonomic garden tools can be the difference between success and injury. I'll walk you through the most ergonomic tools available in Chapter 6.

Focus on You

GET Fit through Gardening is about YOU: your needs, your health, and your muscles. Traditional gardening is about growing plants. Now, what you grow will become secondary to how you grow. This book is about how you bend, move, and approach the physical components of gardening. I'm not going to teach you how to grow anything—except your muscles.

Get Fit through Gardening maximizes the enjoyment and exercise benefits of gardening. Growing vegetables or flowers or the perfect lawn should never take precedence over your personal well-being—physically and emotionally.

I don't expect anyone to perform every gardening session exactly as I've outlined them. While this program introduces many new motions and movements, and may appear to be very regimented, it's not. The goal here is to enhance your enjoyment of gardening, not diminish it. Even changing your gardening habits a little can have a dramatic impact on your physical health. At the very least, adopting the fundamental concepts in this book will help you reduce back strain so you will be less sore after gardening. Also, your hands will be less calloused as your transition the energy from your arms and hands to your legs and torso. Start slow, do what is comfortable for you, and be consistent.

Gardening is something you can do your entire life. If you start today, just adopting the Stance, alternating between a right and left-handed raking position, and alternating between the six weeding positions will have a significant impact on your health. With time, the *Get Fit through Gardening* concepts will become second nature.

About Get Fit through Gardening

This new health and wellness lifestyle includes all the components of lifelong fitness: fresh fruits and vegetables, stretching, moderate exercise, aerobic activities, and strength-training activities. Even better, it's something that can be shared with family and friends.

It's completely different from virtually every other diet and exercise program. Success is measured in seasons, years, and decades. It's something you want to be doing ten, twenty, or even fifty years from now. You will be gardening to exercise and exercising to garden, and it's all as easy as:

- Adopting the new positions like the Lunge and Weed and the Stance.
- Practicing a few minutes a day until you can perform the full thirty-minute workout.
- Using ergonomic tools that allow a wide-legged raking stance, giving you a low center of gravity.
- Planning your gardening sessions with your needs in mind. While you will be tending your lawn and garden, the emphasis is now on your physical requirements and limitations.

Welcome to *Get Fit through Gardening*. If you're new to concepts like repetitions and sets, the muscle groups and the aerobic model—you're in for a treat. If you're new to gardening, then you'll learn how to transform this age-old hobby into a comprehensive fitness program. Either way, you'll learn something exciting and new.

Common Questions about *Get Fit through Gardening*

This Is an Exercise Book, Not a Gardening Book

THE *GET FIT THROUGH GARDENING* program is just as much of a workout as aerobic training, running, weight lifting, Tae Kwon Do, soccer, or tennis. You probably remember your parents' or grandparents' gardens: the gardens were usually large. It may have taken days to till, cultivate, and rake the soil for planting. Your parents might have spent all day digging and weeding, planning to save money and grow vegetables for a large family. Perhaps your mother canned vegetables. That garden is not the garden I recommend.

It's time to reintroduce gardening as a way to exercise. Whether you're a lifelong gardener or new to it, the concepts and techniques you will find here will inspire you to make the transformation from traditional gardening to *Get Fit through Gardening*. How much or how little of the following programs you adopt is completely up to you. After all, balance is key.

IN TRADITIONAL GARDENING	IN *GET FIT THROUGH GARDENING*
large, unmanageable garden	small, stress-free garden
summer garden	spring, summer, and fall garden
raking right-handed	alternating between a right-handed and left-handed stance
one stance per motion	varies between six ways of weeding and multiple standing stances
grows fruits and vegetables for survival	grows fruits, vegetables, and herbs for fun
four to eight hours in one day	short, intense sessions of 5–10 minutes, totaling thirty to sixty minutes, at least three days a week
heavy workouts	light workouts
repetitive use of same muscles	varies garden tasks to exercise many different muscles

Fitness is not a sprint—it's a marathon. As the seasons and years pass, not only will you see the difference in yourself and feel better, you will see the fruits of your labor in magnificent perennial gardens, easy-blooming annuals, and fresh herbs for your table. Every year the fresh fruits and vegetable you grow represent thousands of expended calories. What's not to love?

Never Use the Phrase "Working in the Garden"

From this day forward, never refer to gardening as "work" or "a chore." This simple trick will help you take the first step to transforming traditional gardening into something new and exciting—*Get Fit through Gardening*. Nobody goes to the spa for "aerobic class chores," or practices "soccer chores." Substitute the phrases "gardening exercise" and "exercising in the garden."

Cross-Training Is Encouraged

Cross-training is great to have both during the gardening season and the off-season. What you find in these pages is not a one-stop exercise program. *Get Fit through Gardening* will add new ways to broaden your exercise program and even more importantly, a new way of looking at gardening. There are a number of good, cross-training activities you can do during the off-season or when the weather is not suitable for gardening. I suggest:

- martial arts
- Tai Chi
- dancing (salsa dancing for an exciting change of pace)
- yoga
- Pilates
- walking
- swimming
- aerobics

Use Get Fit through Gardening *with Any Diet Program*

It doesn't matter what diet program you want to follow: Atkins, the Zone, Dean Ornish or Weight Watchers. No diet program will limit the amount of leafy green vegetables, fruits, tomatoes, peppers, eggplant, and fresh herbs you can eat. There is no better way to encourage people to eat more fruits and vegetables than growing them yourself, and exercising in the process!

Where the Idea Came From

I first began to look at gardening as an exercise program when I had young children at home and I found myself unable to go to the gym to work out. At the time, I was actively involved with a local organic gardening network. Organic gardening is more physical than traditional gardening. For example, instead of purchasing a 50-pound bag of chemical fertilizer, an organic gardener adopts a long-term approach and adds hundreds of pounds of composted manure, cotton hulls, and greensand to the soil. This long-term, sustainable approach an organic gardener uses on the soil is conceptually the same long-term, sustainable approach I advocate in the fitness program in *Get Fit through Gardening*.

I found myself moving in a way I'd never seen before in gardening, varying motions often from hand-weeding to standing and weeding, digging, cultivating soil, turning compost, and planting seeds. Some might call it ADD (Attention Deficit Disorder) gardening, which is one reason I believe children will enjoy this energetic fast-paced style of gardening. Carrying baskets of corn stalks, digging, and tilling in the garden became my "workout."

I had just started Tae Kwon Do with my six-year-old son and soon discovered I was transferring the motions and techniques I learned in martial arts to the garden. The martial art concepts of flexibility over strength, range of motion, and emphasizing the legs and torso twisting for power, became key components of *Get Fit through Gardening*.

To me, *Get Fit through Gardening* just makes sense. Every day, you are inundated with quick fixes to lose weight and get healthy that are too good to be true. Rip-off diets and exercise programs abound. The *Get Fit through Gardening* workout is real. It's honest. And it works. Even without the amazing exercise benefits, it's fun and rewarding.

WARM up your muscles before you garden for five to ten minutes. Walk around the garden. Sweep the porch. Deadhead flowers. Use a manual lawn aerator. Warming up promotes an increased awareness of your muscles, improved coordination, improved elasticity and contractibility of muscles, and a greater efficiency of the respiratory and cardiovascular systems.

Stretch for five to ten minutes. Stretching will help prevent back strain, reduce muscle soreness and avoid injury.

Work up to your optimal aerobic training zone. This heart rate range is based on your age and general health (see p. 118). While many gardening activities, such as pruning bushes, will never reach this zone, others such as raking, hoeing and digging most certainly can.

Garden at a steady pace using a variety of motions. Plan out your gardening exercise session to include a variety of movements such as raking, mowing, weeding, pruning, and digging. Alternate between them often, every five to ten minutes.

Stretch again after you have thoroughly exercised aerobically with at least twenty minutes total of steady raking, hoeing, weeding, digging, or mowing.

Cool down after your gardening exercise session by walking, picking flowers or vegetables or just enjoying the fruits of your "exercise."

It's Not Traditional Gardening

Get Fit through Gardening transforms your backyard garden into your own personal gym. Each of the stances have been designed to reflect things commonly found in exercise or circuit programs. For example, the Lunge and Weed is the same lunge you would perform in a gym with dumbbells, except now you're lunging to rid your lawn of pesky weeds. Adding permanent structures such as the chin-up bar, dip bar, or a slanted board for sit-ups, helps to round out your workout and physique.

Virtually every movement you perform in the garden has a gym equivalent. For example, pressing down on a manual lawn aerator will strengthen both the triceps and the legs similar to cable pull-downs and light squats. Adding grip handles to your rake or scuffle hoe will increase the use of your biceps and inner forearm, similar to using dumbbell curls and rotating your arm as you lower the weight.

In addition, gardening motions use a wide variety of primary and secondary stabilizer muscles to perform complex movements that depend on and develop your core strength. This is a tremendous advantage over most exercise machines in your local gym, which work in a restricted plane of motion.

The emphasis on stretching both before and after gardening is sound fitness advice whether you're running a marathon, getting ready to hike, or are preparing for a soccer game—except now you're stretching before and after you garden.

When you move rapidly through different gardening movements (kneeling, squatting, standing, raking, and digging) the *Get Fit through Gardening* program puts you though circuit training, gardening-style. Key concepts like alternating between a right- and left-hand raking stance or using a hand weeder in both your right and left hand will isolate and strengthen muscles on both sides. As you exercise different muscle groups,

12

you'll transform an anaerobic resistance-training exercise into an aerobic one.

With *Get Fit through Gardening*, you're not competing with anyone—except nature and yourself.

Research on Gardening as Exercise

Most experts agree that gardening is a good source of light to moderate exercise. Even literature from the Surgeon General includes gardening as a healthy activity. All research shows that eating fresh fruits and vegetables, exercising moderately and relieving stress is good for you. *The Compendium of Physical Activities Tracking Guide* (Barbara Ainsworth, Arizona State University), lists MET levels for gardening and other common exercises as follows:

MET	ACTIVITY
1.0	Resting quietly
3.0	Walking, 2.5 mph, level, firm surface
4.0	Sweeping garage, sidewalk or outside of house
4.0	Gardening General
4.3	Raking lawn
4.5	Planting trees
4.5	Weeding, cultivating garden
5.0	Clearing land, hauling branches, wheelbarrow chores
5.0	Digging, spading filling garden, composting
6.0	Mowing lawn, walk, hand mower
6.0	Shoveling, light (less than 10 pounds/minute)
6.3	Walking, 4.5 mph, level, firm surface, very brisk
7.0	Shoveling, moderate (10—15 pounds/minute)
8.0	Bicycling, 12—13.9 mph, moderate effort
8.5	Shoveling, digging ditches
9.0	Shoveling, heavy (more than 16 pounds/minute)
10.0	Running, 6 mph (10 minute mile)
10.0	Swimming, laps, freestyle, vigorous effort

MET stands for Metabolic Equivalent and is defined as the ratio of the work metabolic rate to the resting metabolic rate. One MET is the rate at which adults burn a calorie at rest. All activities that have MET values close to 1 are considered sedentary activities.

Activities with values of 3 to 6 METs are considered moderate exercise and will have significant health benefits versus a sedentary lifestyle. Most research illustrates that the greatest health benefits are achieved by adding moderate exercise to a sedentary lifestyle.

Garden to Exercise

THIS program performs one activity to accomplish another. If you plant twenty trees, and ten die, that's okay. You've exercised your body and burned lots of calories.

How Many Calories Will I Burn Gardening?

This question is not that simple to answer because gardening techniques vary widely. It's a lot easier to measure someone running, cycling, or swimming since you can measure steps, strides, or revolutions per minute. The best answer is: it depends. The exact number of calories burned per hour depends on:

- gender
- weight
- Body Mass Index (how muscular you are)
- gardening "technique" and form

- intensity of gardening (repetitions and sets)
- what you are doing (turning compost or digging holes is much more vigorous than planting seeds)

For an 180-lb man, the key *Get Fit through Gardening* activities will burn between 400 to 500 calories per hour. Sustaining a steady rhythm of raking or digging will increase your heart rate. As a general rule of thumb you should be breathing hard but not "out of breath," where you cannot hold a conversation.

Calories Burned During Common Gardening Activities

The following chart gives the calories burned during one hour for a 125-pound woman and an 180-pound man. These numbers apply to traditional gardening stances and techniques. Using *Get Fit through Gardening* stances and techniques and emphasizing the legs and torso versus the arms and shoulders should increase calorie expenditure by 25% to 50%.

Make Your Garden Smaller—Not Larger

KEEP your garden and your yard small so that gardening never feels like work. We don't want gardening to interfere with any of your other hobbies, such as golf, fishing or camping.

Plan your garden so you plant bed one in April, bed two in May, bed three in June, and so on. Add garden beds only after you determine you enjoy *Get Fit through Gardening* and need more exercise (or fresh vegetables for your table).

ACTIVITY	CALORIES PER HOUR (125-POUND WOMAN)	CALORIES PER HOUR (180-POUND MAN)
Gardening General	227	327
Raking lawn	244	352
Planting trees	256	368
Weeding, cultivating garden	256	368
Clearing land, hauling branches, wheelbarrow chores	284	409
Digging, spading, filling garden, composting	284	409
Mowing lawn, walk, hand mower	341	491
Shoveling, light (less than 10 pounds/minute)	341	491
Shoveling, moderate (10—15 pounds/minute)	398	573
Shoveling, digging ditches	483	696
Shoveling, heavy (more than 16 pounds/minute)	511	736

Won't Doing the Lunge and Weed
Ruin the Enjoyment of Gardening?

Using the techniques in this book should enhance, rather than detract from, your enjoyment. They will reduce your back strain and muscle soreness, and add to the aerobic benefits of gardening. While some of these techniques will be awkward at first, after you practice them, they will become second nature. While these stretches and movements are new to you now, they won't be forever. The key is patience, repetition, and consistency. And you don't need to try to do everything in this book for this program to succeed for you. Just add those ideas that make sense to you and add techniques as you master the basics.

I Already Know How to Garden. What's the Big Deal?

Most gardeners move incorrectly as they garden. Most bend over from their back, use only their arms and shoulders, and garden too long using a singular motion or stance. Gardening by itself is not good for you; it's only when you garden using proper form and technique that you reap its benefits. Gardening incorrectly can strain your back and hurt your body, and leave you sore and aching.

Can You Just Garden and
Really Improve Your Health And Lose Inches?

For an optimal workout, you will need to add stretching and resistance training (also known as strength or weight training) to your gardening workout. That's what I've done in the *Get Fit through Gardening* program. This is also true of many good aerobic activities such as running, cycling, and stair-stepping. Also in this book are structures and anaerobic (resistance-training) exercises for those interested in increasing muscle mass and getting a complete workout. For most people, simply adding the improved stances and techniques will be a great workout.

If Gardening Is Good Exercise, Why Don't Gardeners Look Like Bodybuilders?

A lot of gardeners have bad dietary habits. Frying food, eating too many starchy vegetables like beans and corn, and eating a lot of beef and pork can add excessive calories. Portion control is also one of the major reasons for obesity in America today. Whether you're at a restaurant or at the dinner table, there's just too much food on the plate. If one wants to look like a bodybuilder and maintain a body fat ratio under 10%, you need both good genetics and the strictest diet possible in terms of fat and caloric intake.

Garden for Shorter Periods—Not Longer

FOR many of us, it's common to garden all weekend and not quit until the job is done. For optimal aerobic and health benefits I advocate gardening at least three times a week for shorter periods (one to two hours total, alternating activities every 5–10 minutes), and purposely leaving beds unfinished. If you must garden longer than two hours, I purposely decrease the intensity level. Many activities, like repotting plants, are not aerobic, so just cool down and enjoy them. But within a longer gardening session, plan at least one 20-minute session where you reach your optimal aerobic training zone.

If you're looking to significantly increase the size of your muscles, you need to add a resistance-training element to your workout, which gardening just doesn't provide. Even the most strenuous *Get Fit through Gardening* activities, such as digging, double-digging, hoeing, and turning compost will only increase the size of your muscles so much. If, after following the *Get Fit through Gardening* techniques for several seasons, you find yourself wanting more, I highly recommend visiting your local library or bookstore and reading the numerous books on bodybuilding and strength training. I've been "lifting weights" since I was 14 and feel it dramatically improves my overall level of fitness.

If your goal is to lose significant body fat with the *Get Fit through Gardening* workout, you'll also need to focus on your diet. Let's briefly look at some of the most common recommendations for reducing your body-fat ratio:

- Reduce your intake of fat, sugar and starchy foods.
- Eat six small meals each day instead of three large meals.
- Portions of meat, poultry or fish should be about the size of a deck of cards.
- Drink at least eight glasses of water per day.
- Keep a journal and measure everything—what you eat, your physical measurements, your exercise program, and the intensity.
- Set specific goals and time limits (Example: I will lose two inches on my waist by June 8).

How Can I Change Now?

The key here is to change your bad habits. Read through the different suggestions in this book and try the ones that make sense to you. Don't try to do everything at once. Regardless of your age, begin your new stretching regimen today. The benefits of learning this new way of gardening are worthwhile.

19

I Told My Doctor about Get Fit through Gardening

Those unfamiliar with the details will most certainly not understand *Get Fit through Gardening*. Bring a copy of this book and show it to your doctor. Many might think it's a silly idea and that you would only end up hurting your knees and back. In actuality, following this program will decrease the probability of hurting yourself while gardening. Your doctor is thinking about how most people garden and not the specific recommendations of *Get Fit through Gardening*. Ask your doctor if he stretches both before and after gardening, alternates between six different weeding positions every ten minutes, rakes with both a right-handed and left-handed stance, never bends from his back, and wears a heart-rate monitor while gardening. I think he will get the point that this is not a traditional gardening program.

Most doctors advise their patients to change their lifestyle, eat fresh fruits and vegetables, and exercise moderately three times a week. *Get Fit through Gardening* is exactly that. It's preventive medicine and a wellness program. Hopefully, it will also help you to visit the doctor less.

What Do I Do During the Fall and Winter?

Many exercise activities, such as cycling, swimming and running are not suitable during inclement weather (unless you have access to an indoor facility.) Here are some suggestions for off-season activities:

- Use a greenhouse.
- Rake leaves (one or two hours max).
- Plant perennial bulbs.
- Cut firewood.

- Clear brush.
- Plant a fall, winter, or early spring garden.
- Join a garden club.
- Clean your house using the same stance and same leg-bending techniques with a broom or mop.

A Note to Professional Gardeners and Landscapers

IF digging, planting, and raking is part of your livelihood, adopting these techniques will help reduce muscle soreness and back strain. Some of my recommendations, such as making your garden smaller and gardening for short, intense sessions, won't be possible. You're gardening every day, all day, and don't have the luxury of quitting when you feel tired. There are things you can do to help balance the muscles you use and reduce soreness, including:

- Alternate activities or tools every 20 or 30 minutes
- Stretch before and during your workday
- Use your legs and not your back, and never bend from your back
- Use the Stance whenever possible
- Rake, hoe, and weed using a pulling/pushing motion, not a chopping motion

Just adopting a few of these recommendations will help increase your enjoyment of your job.

Ergonomic Tools

2

PURCHASING ERGONOMIC TOOLS or disposing of poorly designed tools, along with adopting the concepts or new gardening motions, will make a significant difference in your gardening experience. Your body will thank you. If you're a gardening professional, using ergonomic tools will help you accomplish more, and work longer, with less risk of injury.

Most garden tools are not designed to minimize your back strain, maximize range of motion, and maximize cutting angle—even though they should be. If your handle is too short (under 57 inches), you cannot adopt the Stance and your full range of motion is limited. The good news is that there are better tools available than there were even five years ago. The bad news: you may have to replace some of your current tools. Consider letting your children use them or donating them to a children's gardening program.

Keep Your Tools Razor Sharp: The Grinding Wheel

Your most important tool is not a garden tool at all, but a grinding wheel to sharpen your tools. I recommend sharpening tools often, at least once a month and more if you use the tool often or in rocky soil. Always keep your garden tools razor sharp. While we want to work up a sweat, we also want the most efficient weeding tool.

Add A Grip Handle To Your Long-Handled Tool

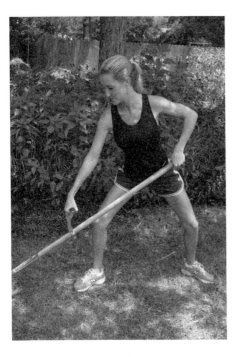

When shopping for ergonomic gardening tools, ask yourself these questions:

- Is the handle long enough to rake or hoe without bending over from your back?
- Does the handle have a grip, or is there an attached hand grip?
- Does the handle have cushioning to minimize calluses?
- Can you use the tool in a pushing/pulling motion?

Avoid tools that can only be used with an up-and-down chopping motion, such as the traditional hoe with a blade at a 90-degree angle. A better tool is one angled at a 45-degree angle, or flat to slice weeds at the soil line as you pull the hoe towards you.

Keep a variety of tools: long-handled tools, hand tools, heavy tools (such as hand mattocks), and light hand tools (Forged Handy Weeder from A.M. Leonard).

Several manufacturers sell handles you can bolt onto your rake or hoe. I highly recommend adding one or more of these to your long-handled tools. They increase your grip, reduce calluses from your hand rubbing up and down on the handle, and increase your raking power.

Standing Tools

Shovels, rakes, and hoes are not the only long-handled tools. There are several types of tools used from a standing position, such as a pitchfork or lawn aerator. Remember, when using any of these tools you should never bend over from your back.

Two garden tools, the Garden Weasel and the Garden Claw, are sold as ergonomic tools. The Garden Weasel has multiple tines and is used in a push/pulling motion. The Garden Claw Cultivator aerates the soil by pressing down and twisting handle. While they might appear to be good, ergonomic tools, unfortunately the handles are much too short for an average-size person. There is no way to use the Garden Weasel in the Stance position and it's difficult to get your hips into the Garden Claw. I don't recommend them, but if you must use them, do so for only very short periods, or look into adding a longer handle.

The Wrist Saver Claw is a good example of ergonomic tool design. Its unique design distributes stress differently and causes the user to garden differently than with a traditional hand cultivator. You use a pulling motion and can dig harder and press down deeper with this tool. It is distributed by Garden Brand of Tools.

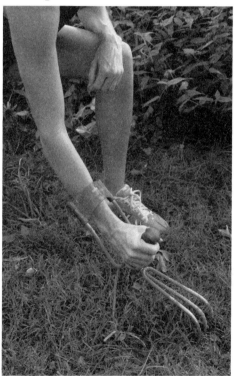

Wrist Saver Claw

USE tools that are pulled and pushed, like a scuffle hoe, which slices the earth as you pull it, versus a traditional hoe that's primarily used in a chopping and pulling motion. If you use a traditional hoe, be sure to rock your body and move your feet as you hoe and focus on the pulling motion versus the up and down chopping motion. Keep your hoeing sessions short—five to ten minutes at most, if possible. If you must hoe for longer periods, then at least take a break or change positions every five to ten minutes.

Recommended Hand Tools: Light

A good example of a user-friendly hand tool is the Forged Handy Weeder by A. M. Leonard. Every gardener should own

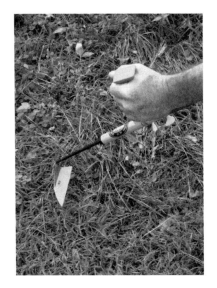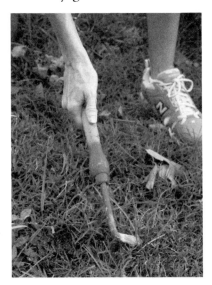

one. This is my number one hand-weeding tool. The razor-sharp, thin blade is perfectly angled for digging or slicing weeds at their base. The tool is used in a push/pull motion as appears in the Lunge and Weed.

The Cape Cod Weeder is another useful L-shaped tool on a short handle. It's useful for digging out weeds and loosening soil between plants and is sturdy with a thick blade. Because of the angle of the blade it does not facilitate the same pulling motion of the Forged Handy Weeder but is a useful tool for working edges.

Recommended Hand Tools: Heavy

V & B Manufacturing has a line of cutting and digging hand tools that include the Hand Mattock. Their six-in-one kit has interchangeable heads and is good for digging out large weeds, shrubs and small trees. This tool is much heavier than the Forged Handy Weeder and the motion and use is different. It's used in more of a swinging motion than a pulling motion. They also have models with different length handles. This tool can be used from the Lunge and Weed stance.

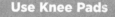

Use Knee Pads

KNEE pads reinforce the kneeling positions and make it more comfortable on your knees.

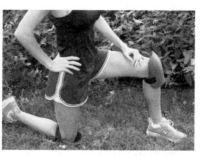

Recommended Flat Blade Hoes

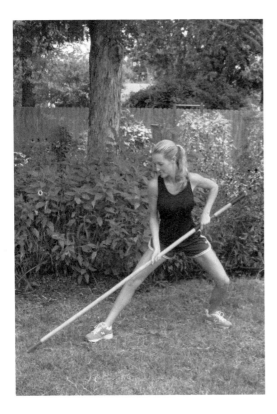

Flat blade hoes are not used in a chopping motion but instead are pulled and pushed. The Heart Hoe featured throughout this book has both a flat, sharp blade as well as an extendable handle that reaches a full six feet. You can also remove the flat blade and use a blade with steel tines called the "Ripper" which literally rips out weeds by the roots as you pull it towards you. The Action Hoe has a sharp, hinged blade that is ideal for the pushing/pulling motion used in *Get Fit through Gardening*. The swan-neck hoe has a long, flat angled blade. Slicing hoes are available from Gardeners Supply, Garden Ease, and Ames/True Temper.

A thin blade is best. Keep the blade razor sharp. Be sure to purchase one with a long handle that can accommodate the Stance position. While some advertisers promote the light weight of their tool, remember that a heavier tool is actually better, because you'll be able to dig deeper into the dirt.

The Mini-Tiller Shuffle

Mini-tillers are lightweight, labor-saving devices useful for areas too small for the larger, traditional tillers. They are light enough for women and senior citizens to pick up and maneuver in narrow, raised beds.

Mini-tillers are operated in a back-and-forth motion as you walk backward, in a motion I've dubbed the "Mini-Tiller Shuffle." This pulling motion exercises the arms, legs, and back muscles. Keep a bend in your legs and use both your arms and legs as you move backward.

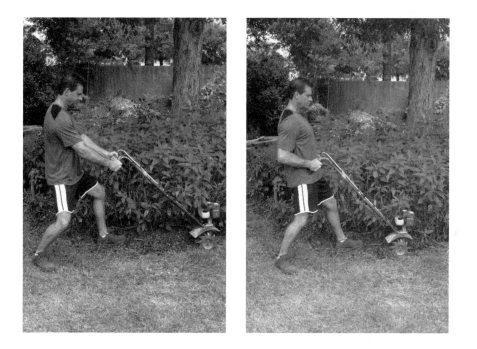

Use a Manual Push Mower

With a manual push mower, you will burn more calories, save on fuel, and avoid the fumes and noise of a power mower. I have a small yard and use a manual mower, but rarely cut both the front and back on the same day. Once a week, I spend fifteen minutes of my workout manually mowing the lawn. Since it's so quiet, it's much more relaxing than a power mower.

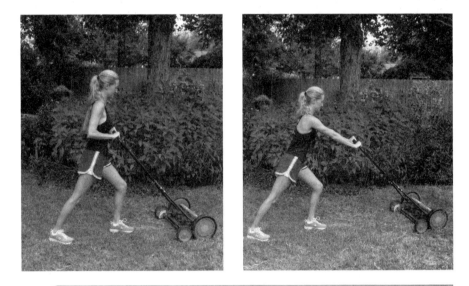

Which is better: A Manual or Power Mower?

A manual mower will burn more calories than a self-propelled one. If your yard is small enough, a manual mower is both environmentally safe and offers more resistance. In addition, with a manual mower, it's much quieter (you can mow early in the morning without bothering your neighbors) and there are no noxious fumes to inhale.

How to Stretch

3

STRETCHING BEFORE GARDENING is often overlooked. While you aren't expected to perform every stretching exercise listed, spending five to ten minutes stretching before every *Get Fit through Gardening* session should become a habit. Your body will thank you.

These are the same stretches you should do for any whole-body activity. The *Get Fit through Gardening* program is designed to transition from traditional gardening, where you primarily use your arms, to primarily using your legs and torso.

Flexibility is a key component of good physical health. Traditional gardening motions often cause us to bend improperly. Therefore, a sound, stretching program is essential. The benefits of stretching are many:

- Enhances overall physical fitness
- Increases mental and physical relaxation
- Promotes awareness of your body
- Reduces risk of a joint sprain or muscle strain

- Reduces muscle soreness
- Reduces muscular tension
- Increases range of motion
- Increases performance of body movements

Stretching Checklist

- Warm up for five minutes before stretching.

- Always stretch slowly.

- Hold the stretch for about fifteen seconds.

- It's best to exhale as you first extend the stretch but inhale and exhale normally while in the stretch.

- Focus on the muscle group being stretched.

- It's best to stretch both before your workout and after.

- Stop stretching if you experience a sharp, acute pain.

- Don't stretch if you've had a recent sprain or strain.

- Don't stretch when you're overly tired. This can lead to injury.

Stretching Program Overview

Ideally, stretching should be done after you've first warmed-up your muscles for five to ten minutes by walking, picking up debris, or sweeping the porch. Warming up means just that: you raise your core body temperature by 1.4 to 2.8 degrees Fahrenheit. Don't stretch before you warm your muscles up.

After stretching, you'll proceed with your *Get Fit through*

Gardening workout, and then stretch again before you cool down. Don't strain, jerk, or bounce while stretching. Slowly and gently stretch your muscles.

There are numerous cool-down gardening activities, like repotting plants, planting seeds and picking or deadheading flowers. Cooling down helps to return your heart rate, breathing and blood pressure to normal. Warming up, stretching, and cooling down improves flexibility and reduces the risk of injury. Also, cooling down removes waste products (lactic acid) from muscle tissue and helps to reduce muscle soreness.

Bending or crouching abruptly or incorrectly while gardening can cause tears of the cruciate ligaments of the knee. Gardening incorrectly can cause injury. One of the main objectives of *Get Fit through Gardening* is to avoid injury while gardening. I cannot overemphasize the importance of gentle stretching. Hold the position for about ten seconds while gently inhaling and exhaling. Never rock or jerk into a stretch. Repeat the stretching process several times.

In particular, you should stretch the Achilles tendon (the tendon in the lower back part of your ankle), the abductors and adductor muscles of the groin, and the ligaments and tendons of the thigh (quadriceps) muscles. For those inspired by the concept of *Get Fit through Gardening*, I recommend adding yoga, Tai Chi or Pilates classes to your weekly workouts. If you're ambitious try a martial art like Tae Kwon Do or karate.

35

Stretch the Muscles in Your Inner Thigh and Groin

The cornerstone movements of the *Get Fit through Gardening* workout are the raking Stance and the Lunge and Weed. These bent-knee, wide-legged, low-center-of-gravity stances will naturally stretch your groin. These movements are crucial to improving the exercise benefits of your gardening. Take your time (and by that I mean weeks and months) to gently stretch into these positions each gardening session.

Basic Types of Stretches

Stretches are either dynamic (involving motion) or static (involve no motion). Before you garden, it's best to do dynamic stretches and static stretches. Dynamic stretches use movement to stretch and loosen your muscles and consist of controlled leg and arm movement that will take you slowly and gently to the limits of your range of motion. Be careful to not perform any bouncing or jerking movements. Dynamic stretching should be performed in sets of eight to twelve repetitions. Examples of dynamic stretching include slow, controlled:

- Arm swings
- Torso twists
- Toe touches

Static stretching is also referred to as relaxed stretching or passive stretching. Many commonly known stretches are static. In a static stretch, you assume a position and hold it with some other part of your body, or with the assistance of a partner, the ground, or a device. Examples of static stretching include most of the basic stretches listed in this book.

36

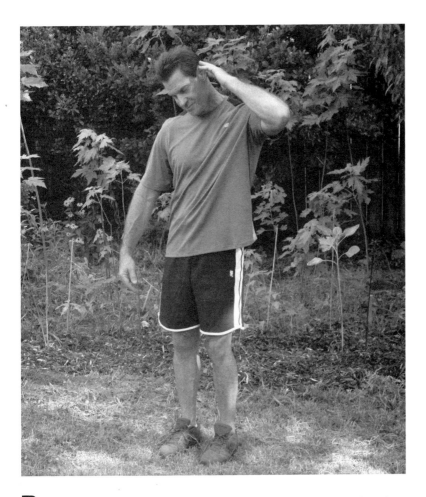

Roll your neck gently in a circle. Use your opposite hand to push gently down for a thorough stretch, and remember, stop if you ever feel pain. Exhale and inhale deeply as you stretch your neck.

Wrist Stretch

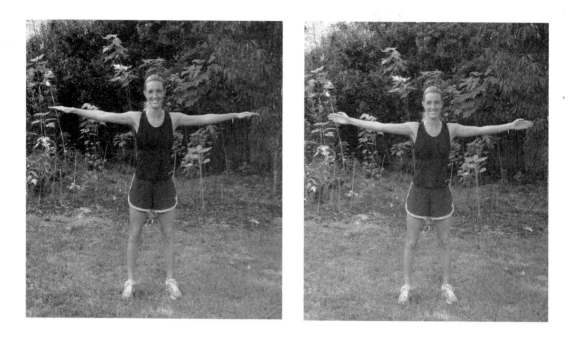

Gently hold out your arms in front of you. Stand with your back straight and gently shake both hands up and down at the wrist. You can perform this stretch several times during the duration of your exercise, not just before it. Try it after hand-weeding or digging with a trowel.

38

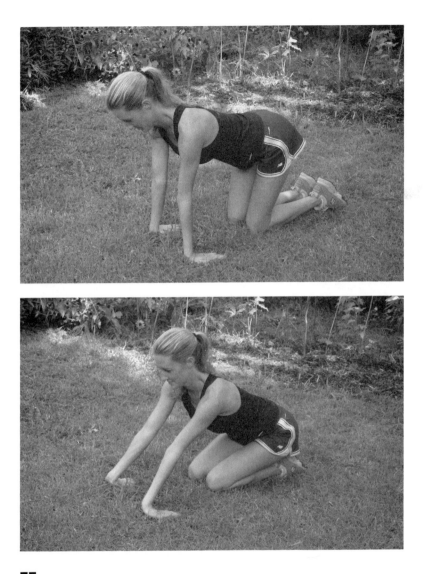

Kneel on the grass or a mat. Place your palms flat on the ground, with your fingers pointing back towards your knees. Gently lean backwards, keeping your palms flat on the floor. You should feel mild tension through your wrists and forearms. Exhale and hold this stretch for 5 to 10 seconds.

Arm Rotations

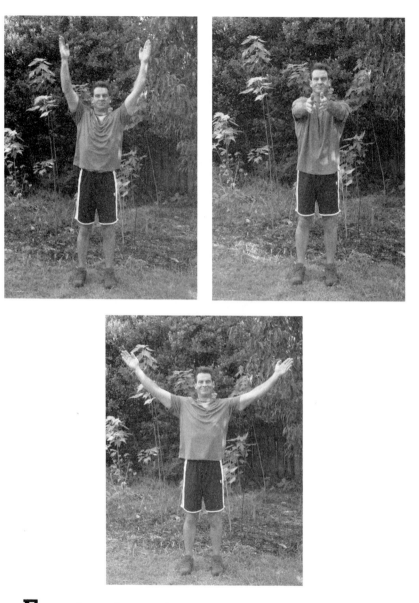

For an immediate pick-me-up, swing your arms in a circle around your torso. Do not swing wildly; this should be controlled. Try for 10 to 15 rotations to get the blood pumping.

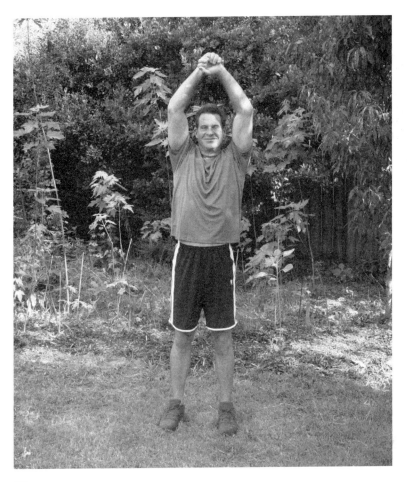

Sit or stand upright. Cross one wrist over the other and inter-lock your hands. Inhale, straighten your arms, and extend your arms up over your head. Your elbows should be behind your ears. Hold the stretch, relax, and return your hands to a 90-degree position relative to your body.

Toe Touch

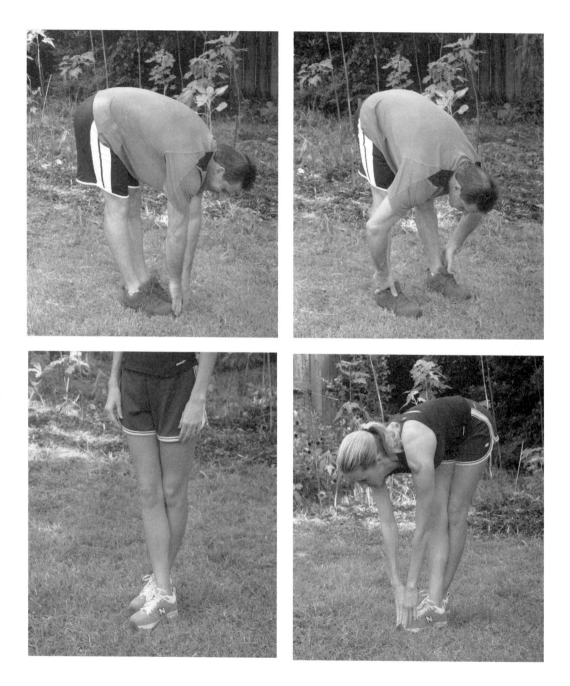

Slowly bend over from the waist and touch your toes. Don't jerk or bounce but gently ease into the stretch. Exhale as you stretch down. Inhale as you return to an upright position. For a greater stretch of the Achilles tendon, cross your feet at the ankles and bend over to touch your toes. When you first attempt this stretch you may want a pole or stand nearby for balance.

If you are unable to touch your toes or have not done this for many years, I would recommend the sitting or supported stretches first.

Shoulders Stretch

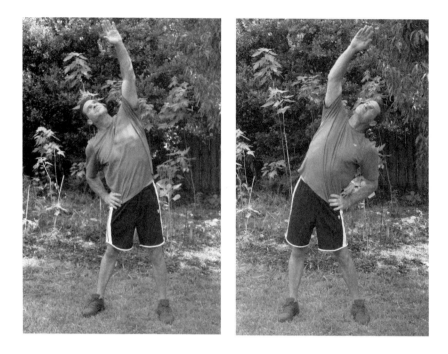

From either a sitting or standing position, set your shoulders square and reach across your body with your right arm. With your left hand holding your right arm just beyond your elbow, press your right arm closer in to your body, until you feel a mild tension in your shoulder. Exhale and hold the stretch for 5 to 10 seconds. Repeat this stretch on your opposite side.

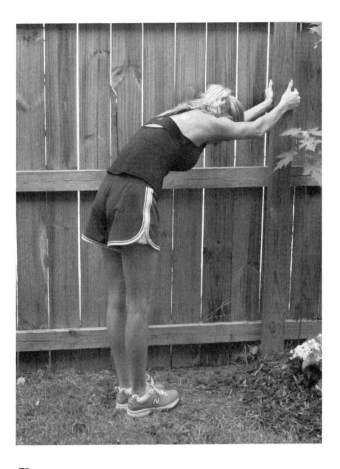

Stand upright with your feet together about 3 feet from a tree or wall. While keeping your arms and legs straight, flex at your waist, flatten your back, and grasp the supporting surface with both hands. Extend your shoulders, and press down on the supporting surface to produce an arch in your back. Exhale and hold the stretch for 5 to 10 seconds.

Torso Twists

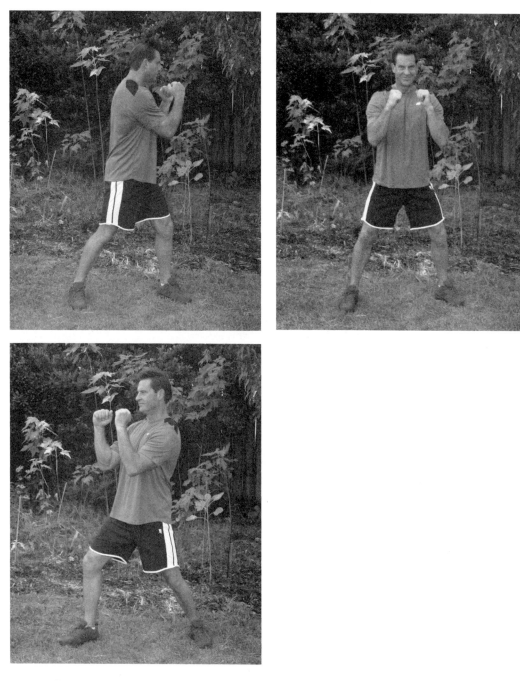

Stand straight with your arms in front of you in a boxing stance. Twist your torso from side to side and hold the stretch. Maintain a small bend in your knees.

Alternatively, perform this stretch with a broomstick handle across your shoulders. Be careful not to jerk but stretch slowly, exhaling and inhaling regularly.

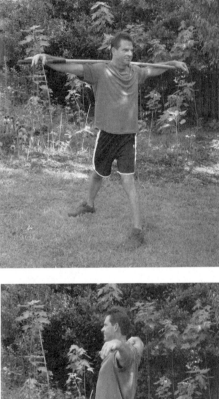

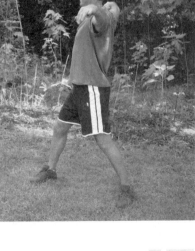

Chest Stretch

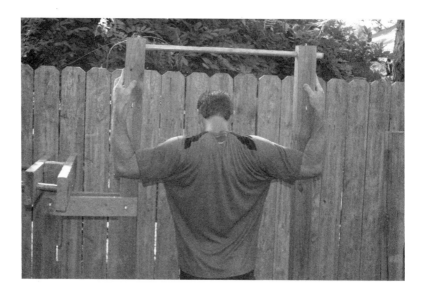

From either a sitting or standing position, extend your arms straight out to the side, with your palms forward. Relax your neck as you press your straight arms back and hold until you feel a mild tension throughout your chest. If you have a chin-up bar, you can use the two chin-up posts to facilitate this stretch. Press against both posts with your hands. You should feel the stretch in your chest. Exhale and hold this stretch for 5 to 10 seconds.

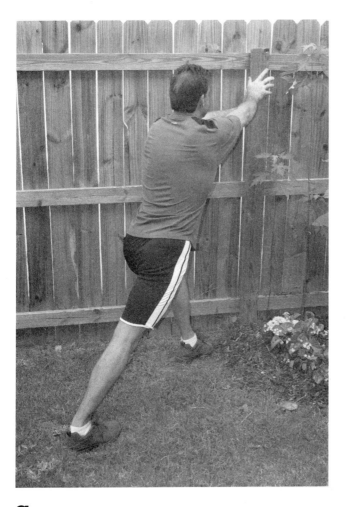

Stand upright four or five steps from a tree or pole. Bend one leg forward and keep your opposite leg straight. Lean against the tree without losing the straight line of your head, neck, spine, pelvis, outstretched leg and ankle. Keep your rear foot down, flat and parallel to your hips. Exhale, bend your arms, move your chest toward the wall and shift your weight forward. You will feel the stretch in your lower leg (the right leg, in this photo). Exhale and hold the stretch for 5 to 10 seconds.

Hamstrings Stretch

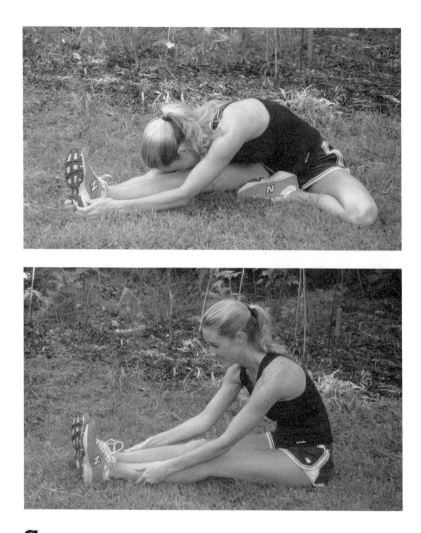

Sit with your right leg stretched out in front of you, toe point-ing up, and your left leg bent in towards you. Bend forward at your hips and lean over your right leg. Exhale while holding this stretch for 5 to 10 seconds, then change legs.

Next, stretch both legs out in front of you, toes pointing up. Bend forward at your hips and lean over your legs. Exhale while holding this stretch for 5 to 10 seconds.

❧ Sitting Quadriceps and Hamstring Stretch

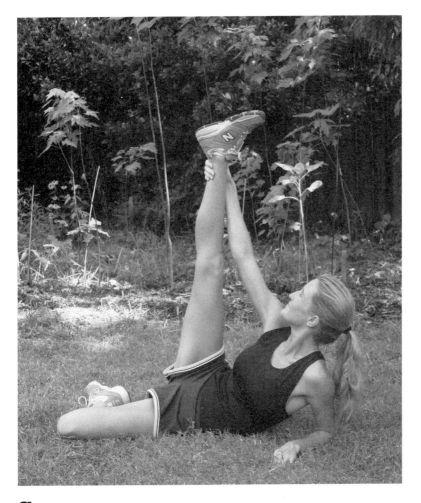

Sit comfortably on the ground or a mat with your legs out-stretched to both sides. Lean to your right side and stretch your left leg straight up, reach out with your left hand, grab your foot (or ankle) and pull your leg back stretching the underside of your lower and upper leg. Exhale as you stretch. Repeat with your right leg.

This is a great stretch, in particular for the *Get Fit through Gardening* motions and stances.

Quadriceps Stretch

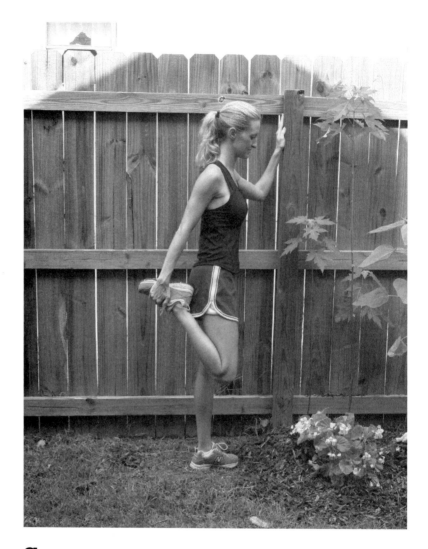

Stand upright with one hand against a tree or a wall for balance. Bend one leg up and raise your foot to your buttocks. Slightly flex the supporting leg. Exhale, reach down, grasp your raised foot with one hand, and pull your heel toward your buttocks without overcompressing the knee. Hold the stretch for 5 to 10 seconds.

EVEN with stretching and the best preparation and technique, it's easy to overdo gardening. If you're sore be sure to follow traditional remedies for muscle soreness.

- ❦ Rubbing compound like Ben-Gay
- ❦ Heating pad
- ❦ Massage
- ❦ Whirlpool Jacuzzi

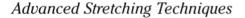

Advanced Stretching Techniques

In addition to stretching by muscle group, and specific stretches, there are many different approaches to stretching. The following are but a sample:

- ❧ Ballistic stretching
- ❧ Dynamic stretching
- ❧ Active stretching
- ❧ Passive (or relaxed) stretching
- ❧ Static stretching
- ❧ Isometric stretching
- ❧ PNF stretching

There are numerous books on advanced stretching. What has been included in this book is sufficient to improve your gardening experience and prepare you for the *Get Fit through Gardening* exercise program. If you are curious or ambitious about advanced stretches, what follows are some different approaches or techniques.

You should warm up before you do active and isometric stretches. Active stretches, also referred to as static stretches, are those where you assume a stretch and hold it with no assistance other than the strength of your agonist muscles. An example would be bringing your leg up high and then holding it there without anything to keep the leg in that extended position. The tension of the agonist muscles in an active stretch helps to relax the muscles being stretched (the antagonists) by reciprocal inhibition. Many of the movements (or stretches) found in various forms of yoga are active stretches.

Isometric stretching, a type of static stretching, involves the resistance of muscle groups through isometric contractions or tensing of the stretched muscles. Isometric stretching is not recommended for children and adolescents with bones still growing.

PNF (Proprioceptive Neuromuscular Facilitation) stretching is an advanced method that can be performed for most major muscle groups. PNF stretches use a series of contractions, done against a partner's resistance, and relaxations. PNF stretches safely stretch beyond the muscle's normal length by pressing in the opposite direction of the stretch. These are best performed with a partner's assistance. This is an advanced stretching technique. I include it because it helped me, after the age of 40, improve my stretching considerably—but that was after performing traditional stretches for two to three years. Before attempting a PNF stretch you should use caution, be familiar with common stretches and be sufficiently warmed up. The Butterfly Stretch is an example of a PNF stretch you can perform without a partner.

I include it because it helped me, after the age of 40, improve my stretching considerably—but that was after performing traditional stretches for two to three years.

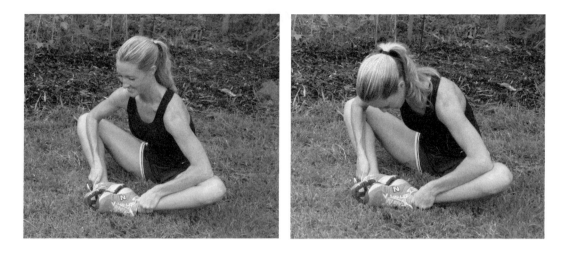

This is a good stretch for the inner thigh muscles. There are two ways to do this stretch. For the traditional butterfly stretch, sit up straight on the grass or a mat, with knees bent, feet close to your body, pressing the bottom of your feet together. Grab your ankles with your hands and place your elbows on your knees. Gently lean your chest forward and press both knees down with your hands. Exhale and hold the stretch for 5 to 10 seconds. Don't rock or bounce.

To do the more advanced PNF version, start in the same seated position with the bottom of your feet together. First, press your knees up against your elbows while pressing down with your arms. Hold this stretch for 15 seconds. Next, gently press both knees down with your arms as you lean forward. Hold this stretch for 15 seconds.

Side Splits Stretch

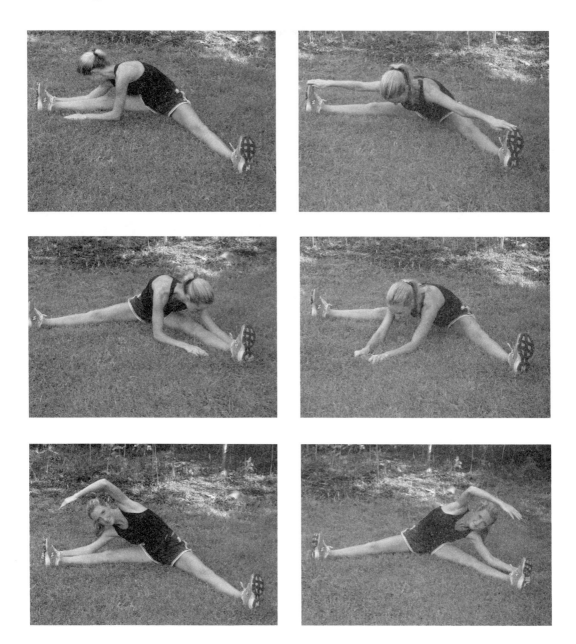

Sit upright on the ground or a mat with both legs straight. Straddle your legs as wide as possible to the sides. Facing front, exhale, rotate your trunk, and extend your upper torso onto your leg. Concentrate on keeping both the lower back and the legs extended. Exhale and hold the stretch for 5 to 10 seconds.

This is a very difficult stretch. Tanya, our model, is very flexible. Don't be discouraged if you can't stretch as far as is shown in these photos. I personally have never achieved a full 90-degree angle and don't expect you to either. Just stretch as far as feels comfortable to you. With practice, you will improve. As in your gardening, your patience and persistence will be rewarded.

The Martial Arts Crescent Kick 🌿

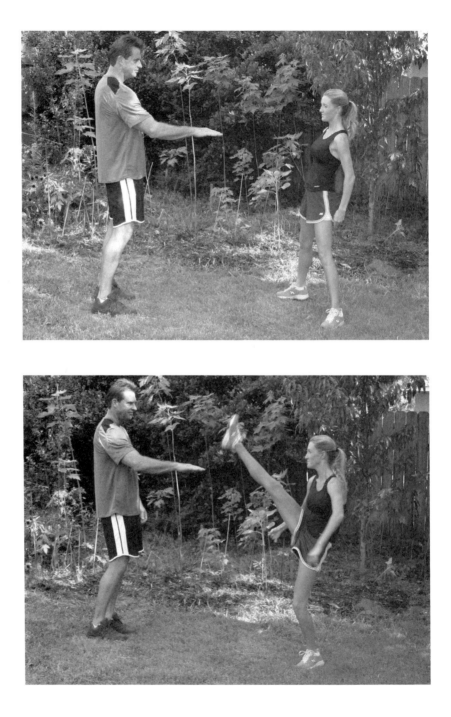

This advanced stretch should only be performed at the end of your warm-up or as part of your post-workout stretching. With just a little practice you will be able to kick much higher than anyone could imagine. The kicking foot first travels inward and then travels outward in an arc. The movement begins as a circular movement traveling inward and upward. At the intended height, the foot travels horizontally and outward, then completing its circular and downward movement back to the ground.

Once you have this movement down, practice kicking leaves on a tree. This will stretch your inner thigh muscles.

Beginners beware: Stretch for at least ten minutes before you attempt the Crescent Kick, and always perform the move in a slow and deliberate manner in a small circle in front of you. Beginners should not kick above waist height. Remember, you're not kicking so much as throwing your leg in an arc. All of the power comes from your hip rotation.

1 Not stretching before and after you weed, dig, or hoe in the garden.

2 Maintaining the same stance (right or left) all day long.

3 Repeating the same weeding, raking or hoeing motion over and over for hours.

4 Raking, hoing, or digging for hours without resting or taking a break.

5 Not preparing properly for early spring gardening. (Ease into it!)

6 Bending from the back and not the knees.

7 Maintaining a yard or garden that is too big for your needs or personal enjoyment.

8 Jerking your rake or hoe with a choppy, up and down motion.

9 Exacerbating a previous back or knee problem using poorly designed, short-handled tools.

10 Holding your breath while you rake, dig, or hoe.

Gardening Motions and Muscles

4

IT'S HARD TO determine which component of *Get Fit through Gardening* is the most important. The easy answer is they are all equal, but ultimately, the actual raking, weeding, and digging motions burn calories and tone your muscles.

Abdominal and Additional Strength Training Exercises

While you will tense and relax your abs during many gardening movements, it's difficult to isolate those muscles as effectively as a simple sit-up or leg lift can. For the gardener who is serious about using their yard as a gym, my recommendations are to purchase an exercise mat and consider our advanced chapter, which includes many simple projects that should only take a hour or two to construct.

A key part of the *Get Fit through Gardening* program is changing your stance and motion often. To these ends, you will adopt many different weeding positions using a trowel, hand weeder, hand-hoe, or hand-rake. While I recommend using a pulling motion, any tool will work as long as long as you keep changing your position every three to five minutes.

Proper Get Fit through Gardening *Attire*

You should always garden with a wide stance, knees over feet, a hand grip, and a long handle. Use a foam mat or kneepads when kneeling. Be comfortable and protect yourself while gardening. Wear gloves, kneepads, and a wide-brimmed hat. Use sunscreen and insect repellent. Have a water bottle available.

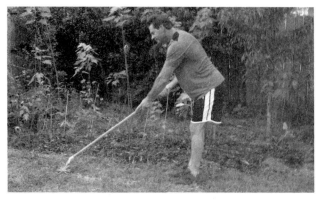

INCORRECT. The handle is too short, he's bending over from the back, he's not wearing a hat or gloves, and his legs are straight.

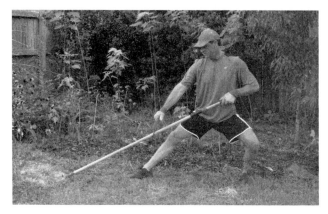

CORRECT. Note the hat, gloves, long handle, hand grip, and the Stance raking technique.

Bad Gardening Technique

The following photographs illustrate bad gardening exercise technique.

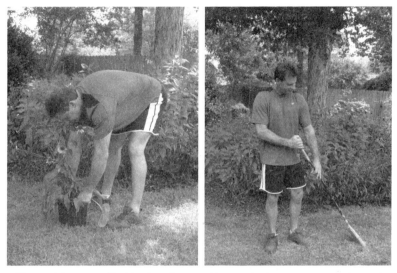

Never pick up a potted bush or tree by bending from back.

Never rake, hoe, or sweep using only your arms with your legs straight.

Good Gardening Technique

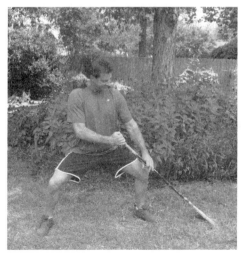

When I advise people to assume a wide-legged stance, they typically spread their feet out but don't bend at the knee and their knee is not over their foot. This splayed-leg stance has little power and can injure your knees. For proper technique, the knees must be bent and the knee is above the foot and the lower leg is vertical as shown in the photo. Always stretch first and gradually assume the correct stance.

The Stance

GYM EXERCISE:
Squat and Row

The Stance works the quadriceps and the gluteus maximus. It's somewhere between doing squats and working a stair-step or elliptical machine. It's a solid, low-impact exercise. It will also stretch the groin so ease into this exercise gently and slowly at first and increase duration and intensity gradually. You will get the most benefit from this exercise in the fall when raking leaves.

The Stance is the most important movement unique to this book. It can be used for a wide variety of activities: sweeping, raking soil, raking leaves, cultivating, and hoeing. This stance is radically different from the way you currently rake or sweep. Instead of using the small muscles of your arms, shoulders, and lower back to rake and hoe, you'll be using the large muscles of your legs and buttocks. In martial arts, this stance position is known as the "horse stance" or "middle stance."

You will need to ease into the Stance gradually, practicing it every day. With its low center of gravity, it will stretch your groin and might be a bit uncomfortable at first. For your first session, practice it for just a few minutes, and for each subsequent session, add a few more minutes. Gradually add time and increase intensity until you feel comfortable with this movement. If all else fails—practice! With steady, constant practice, the Stance will become natural and fun. You won't even be aware you're doing it. If your goal is to lose weight, this motion should be your primary exercise.

1. Remember to warm up and stretch before you attempt this pose. You will need a long-handled rake or hoe to perform this motion. Adding a grip or handle will help you in the pulling motion.
2. Spread your legs wide. Your legs should not be splayed out. In other words, bend your legs at the knees so that your knees are above your feet (The shins are

vertical.) It will look like a half-crouch, like a football player on the line of scrimmage.

3. Feet are parallel and wide; about 1½ shoulder width apart. Point your toes forward. Weight is central and low, with your back straight. You will feel a stretch in your groin.

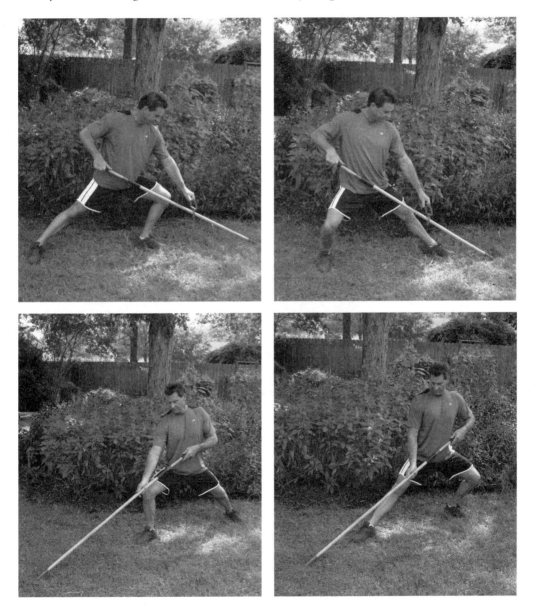

4. Now, rock your body back and forth while scooting your feet side-to-side to rake. Your arms will move relatively little. You will keep your feet stationary and rock your body in the direction of the rake. If you're raking right-handed, your left leg will bend and lower and your body will lean toward the rake. Then your entire body, not just your arms, will rock back. The lower the crouch, the better the workout.

5. As you rake toward yourself, you will move your legs and body more than your arms. Your arms will move some, but the focus and power will come from your lower body.

6. Pay close attention to your breathing and inhale in as you move the rake out from your body and exhale as you pull the rake toward you.

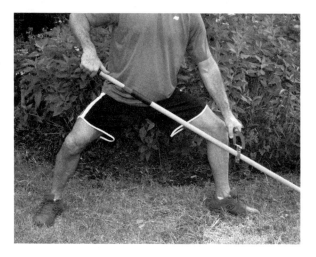

Depending upon your level of fitness, you may find yourself quickly out of breath. You might also feel very conscious of your quadriceps and a stretch in your groin. Since you've never raked this way before, this motion will feel startlingly new. That's all good, but don't overdo it. Rest often at first and rake in bursts of ten to fifteen strokes.

Even if you are right-handed, you should alternate between a right-handed and a left-handed stance. Yes, this will be awkward at first and might slow you down, but you are building up muscles on both sides of your body instead of working only your dominant side.

If you're raking leaves, be sure to move your feet as you rock back. Again, the goal is to move your legs as much as possible and your arms as little as possible.

YOU can use the Stance while sweeping indoors or outdoors with a broom.

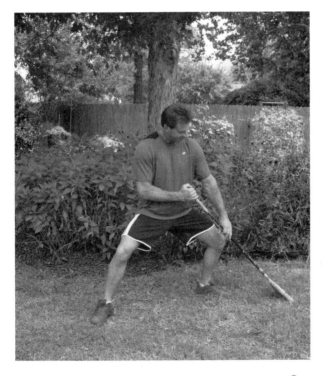

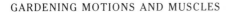

Classic Lunge and Weed 🌿

Compare the gym version of the lunge and the *Get Fit through Gardening* version of the Lunge and Weed. They are essentially the same movement. One is performed indoors in a gym where it seems normal to lunge and walk forward alternating legs while holding light hand weights. The other involves lunging and digging out weeds or crabgrass from your lawn or garden.

A slicing hand tool that you can pull, like the Forged Handy Weeder seen in Chapter 2, is the very best type of tool for this motion. The crouching stance and focus on the legs is very similar to the Stance but you're now bending one leg forward in a lunge instead of out to the side. You might want to use a cart, a stand, or a pitchfork (stab it into the ground next to you) to help keep your balance at first.

1. Stand naturally with the Forged Handy Weeder in your right hand.
2. Lunge with your left leg forward. You should not rest your knee on the ground. Never, ever let your lunging knee move ahead of its foot; this is dangerous.

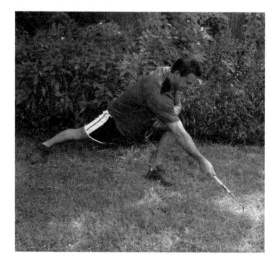

70

3. Rest your left elbow on your left knee as you lunge for balance.
4. Reach out in front of you with your hand-weeder and pull it toward you, slicing the weed at the root.
5. Stand and move to the next spot and repeat the lunging and weeding motions. You can lunge forward to the next spot if you want an extra workout.
6. After 3 to 4 minutes, switch sides.

Once you are able to perform this motion without a balance, increase the speed and how far your trailing leg lowers to the ground.

Lunge and Weed Across the Body ✍

GYM EXERCISE:
The Lunge, Cable
Row, Abdominal
Obliques

A variation of the Lunge and Weed is to squat and pull the weeder across your body. For example, if you are weeding with your right hand, reach far across to the left and pull the blade in front of you in a wide arc, as shown in the photos below.

The key to this motion, as with the many other new motions and techniques in this book, is steady and consistent practice. What may be awkward at first, with practice and repetition will become completely normal.

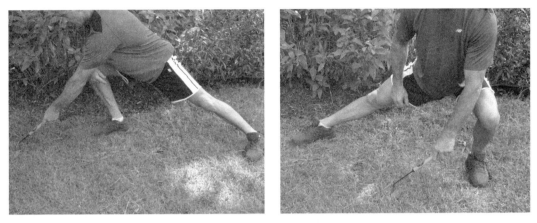

Lunge and Weed Across the Body—Left Hand.
Notice how he rocks from right to left.

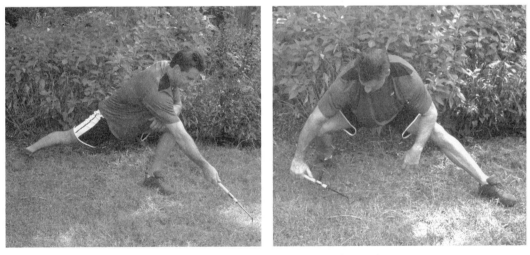

Lunge and Weed Across the Body—Right Hand.

Six Weeding Positions To Prevent Injury

1. The Lunge and Weed

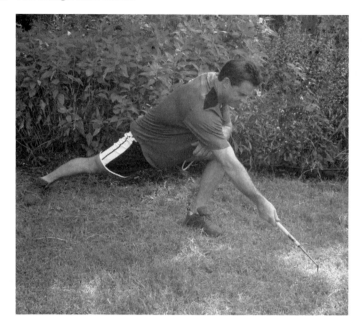

2. One leg bent, other knee on the ground

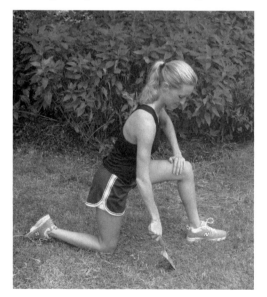

3. Two legs bent kneeling

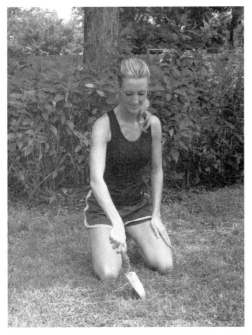

4. Sit and garden

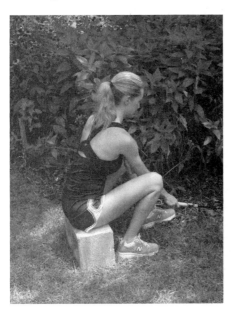

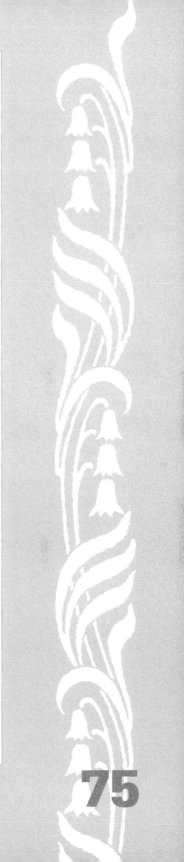

5. Full resting squat and weed

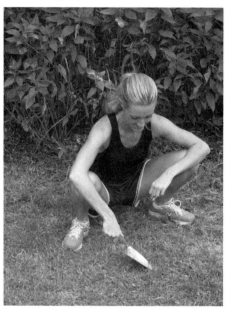

6. The Stance

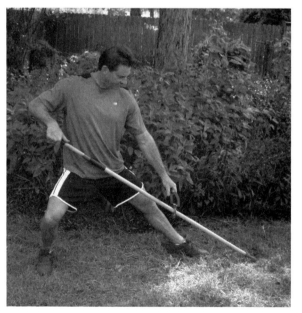

ALTERNATE often between six different gardening positions. Be sure to stand up every five to ten minutes and be sure to alternate legs. Always be sure to stretch before using any of the Lunge and Weed or kneel and weed movements.

Note: The Lunge and Weed and the Stance are dynamic, active positions to get you into shape. The other four positions use primarily your arms and shoulders and will protect your back from injury. They are good positions for elderly gardeners.

1. The Lunge and Weed

Review the directions on page 70.

2. One Leg Bent, Other Knee on the Ground

This kneeling position is best done using knee pads or a soft foam pad. You might want to have a cart or stand nearby to help yourself up at first. Be sure to stand up every five to ten minutes and change positions often.

1. Standing normally, lunge with your left leg, left foot flat on the ground.
2. Bend your right leg so your knee rests on the ground. Rest your left elbow on your left knee for balance.
3. Dig or weed as you would normally.

To get up from this position without harming yourself, try this movement. Pivot and turn your torso from left to right as you move your right leg from a kneeling position to a squatting, wide-hipped position. Stand up.

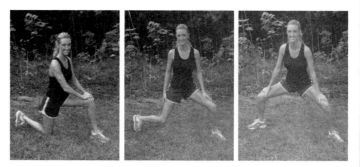

This is a preferred way to stand up if you are carrying a lot of weight or are older. It places less stress on your knees. You might need to use this standing technique several times a day.

3. Two Legs Bent Kneeling

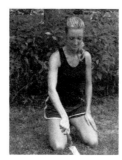

This is a stance to reduce back strain from stooping over. Weed while kneeling with both knees on a pad or using knee pads. Since this stance exercises primarily your arms (and we want you to focus on using your legs), I would recommend it for only short periods of time, a change of pace, or if your knees won't permit other motions. The main focus of this position it to prevent you from bending over and hurting your back. Commercial kneelers are available that both help cushion the knees and provide support when standing up or kneeling down.

4. Sit and Garden

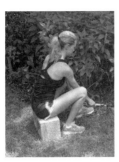

Sitting and gardening is ideal for the cool-down period. Alternate between more strenuous positions and less strenuous ones.

5. Full Resting Squat and Weed
GYM EXERCISE: Weighted squat

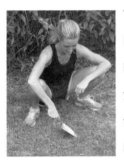

This position is more difficult as we age. For young children a squatting position is quite natural. Stand straight, with your feet pointing at a 45-degree angle from your body, squat with both legs bending at the knees. Stand up every three to five minutes and breathe deeply.

I would assume this position only if your knees permit it and you're sufficiently warmed up. You should bend down slowly and hold the position and weed for only a few minutes at first. If you find this position difficult at first, it will become more comfortable as you increase your stretching both before and after gardening.

6. The Stance

Review the directions on page 66.

Lawnmower In and Out

GYM EXERCISE:
Bench Press

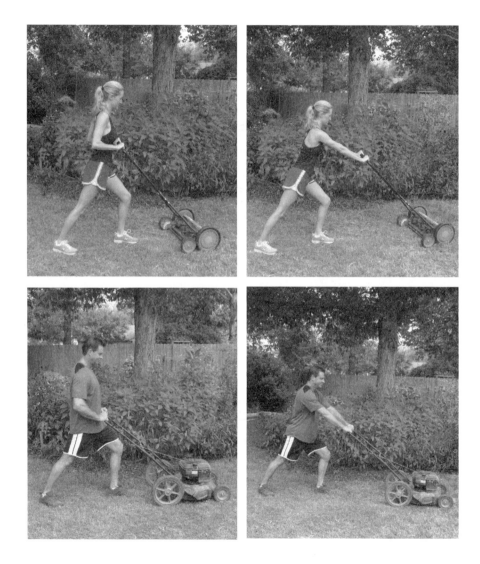

The two most common chest exercises are the push-up and bench-press. In *Get Fit through Gardening,* the equivalent exercise requires a lawnmower. This can either be a regular gas mower or the more environmentally friendly push mower. While this exercise won't strengthen your chest like a bench press with a heavy weight, it will help tone your chest muscles. This exercise won't work with a self-propelled mower and will be much more difficult on a sloped lawn and when the grass bag is full.

1. With a lawnmower in front of you, grasp the handle with both hands and take one step forward but allow your arms to bend at the elbow and the handle (and your hands) to come to your chest.
2. Using your arms, push the lawnmower forward with your arms as if you were bench pressing the mower. This will exercise your chest and triceps. A wide grip will exercise your chest more. A narrow grip will exercise your triceps more.
3. Take another step with your other leg again allowing the handle to meet your chest.
4. Repeat the process, alternating walking and pushing the lawnmower forward.

You need not perform this exercise while mowing your entire lawn or every time you mow, but use it to strengthen the triceps and pectoral muscles.

You have to be pushing out from your chest or moving your arms from the side to the front of your chest to exercise the pectoral muscles.

I would suggest only performing this for 3 to 4 sets of 15. If it takes ½ hour to mow your lawn then perform the chest-push technique for about half the time or about 15 minutes.

Digging

GYM EXERCISE:
Squats and
Lateral Bends

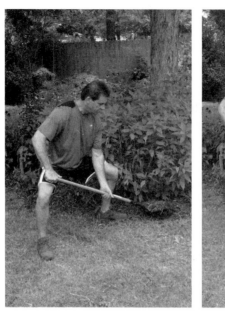

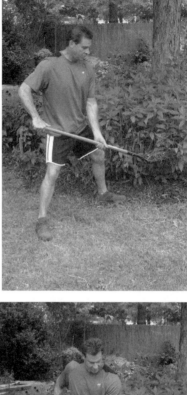

Always strive to lift the dirt using your legs and not just your arms. Keep your knee bent. The first time you use this technique, your legs may be a little sore the next day. That's a sign you're doing it correctly.

82

Most people dig a hole, turn a compost pile, or double-dig using primarily their arms. Instead, you'll focus on your legs and torso. To do this you will bend at your knees and move your entire body, not just your arms.

Everyone knows digging a hole is strenuous exercise. For our purposes, I advise planning your sessions so you can dig no longer than about 20 to 30 minutes total. Unless you're in great shape, or a professional landscaper, avoid digging holes for 2 or more hours at a time. Keep your digging sessions short and within your overall fitness plan.

Practice digging by moving your arms as little as possible. At first this will seem awkward and difficult. But after a while it will become easier, burn more calories, and your arms will not be as sore afterwards. The legs are made up of some of the largest and most powerful muscles in the body.

1. Keep your back straight and push your spade into the soil with your right foot as you would do normally.
2. Now, when pulling up on the soil, adopt a wide stance, bending at your knees.
3. Raise the soil using your legs, not your arms.
4. Twist at your hips and turn your torso, dropping the soil.
5. Repeat, remembering to emphasize and focus on your legs to dig and raise the soil with your back straight.

This is a great back-saving motion. Practice this often. Remember to breathe in and out as you dig and turn. Take a break if you feel winded after 5 to 10 minutes of vigorous digging.

Lawn Aerator

GYM EXERCISE:
Triceps Pull-Down,
Squats

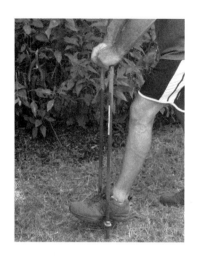

This is a good warm-up activity that requires a manual, multi-pronged lawn aerator tool. You will push down on the bar with your arms, working your triceps, as you alternate your right and left leg. Maintain a steady pace and aerate the soil for 5 to 10 minutes. Soil aerators are particularly good if you have dense clay soil. This simple exercise is a great one for those with limited knee mobility.

1. Raise the lawn aerator out before you and step on the lower rail with your right foot.
2. Push the tines into the ground bending forward using your weight.
3. Rock the tines back and forth (if you have dense, clay soil) as you push.
4. Lift the lawn aerator from the ground with your arms in a fluid motion.
5. Continue moving forward and pushing the tines into the ground.

Alternate this motion with other techniques like the Stance or the Lunge and Weed.

84

✎ The Post-Hole Digger

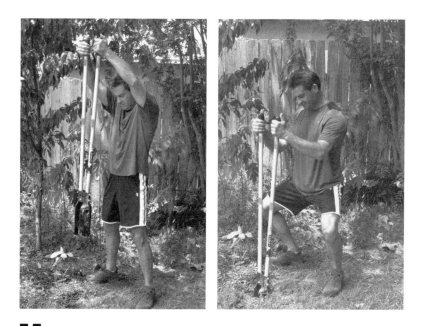

Maintain a bend in your knees and use your legs. I like this exercise because it's a powerful movement using the whole body. Don't overdo it.

1. Hold the post-hole digger in front of you, maintaining a bend in your legs to avoid any strain on your back.
2. Keep your back straight as you raise the post-hole digger up and stab it into the ground.
3. Press the handles together.
4. Using, your legs, raise from a squatting position to a standing position.
5. Twist your body to the side and deposit the soil.
6. Repeat the motion, remembering to alternate twists to the side.

Quit when you are tired or sore. You can use this technique when planting small shrubs or perennials. You can also spot dig in your raised garden bed and fill the hole with compost.

Picking Up Objects ✍

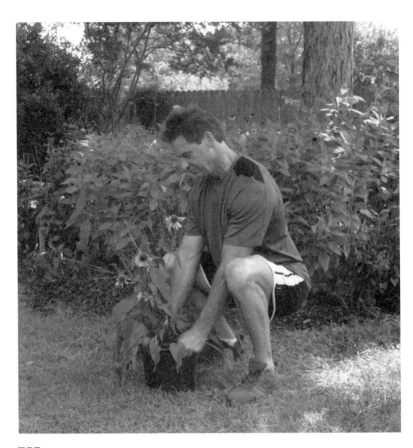

Whether you're picking up a potted bush, a tree, or a bag of soil or mulch, always use your legs, not your back.

1. With the soil bag or potted plant in front of you, keep your back straight as you squat down from the knees.
2. Grasp the soil bag or potted plant and raise straight up using your legs.

Be sure to warm up and stretch before you attempt lifting a series of heavy objects. If the object is heavier than you can lift, use a wheelbarrow, cart, or a hand truck.

86

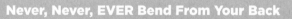

PRUNING trees or bushes could be a warm-up activity or part of your cool-down. It primarily exercises the shoulders and forearms. Use a ratchet pruner if you can find one. It does not require as much hand strength and can cut thicker branches than an anvil type pruner.

Never, Never, EVER Bend From Your Back

WHILE this may sound like common sense, most gardeners bend from their back often—and pay the price. Instead of bending from your back, adopt the Stance, practice the Lunge and Weed, and alternate between the six different gardening positions. Short handled rakes and hoes tools (less than 57 inches) are another major reason people stoop over from their back.

Adding Resistance Training: Structures and Other Exercises

5

ADDING SIMPLE STRUCTURES and traditional strength-training exercises to your *Get Fit through Gardening* workout will transform your backyard into your personal gym. Resistance training will build muscle strength. While some garden activities, such as digging and turning the compost, require significant strength, they will only tone your muscles so far.

While you won't be technically gardening or growing anything, adding these structures to your backyard will provide a natural and organic addition to your workout. These simple structures will help you balance your workout with resistance training, increasing the workout of your stomach, biceps, and pectoral muscles.

Structures can also help when your gardening activities for a particular day don't reach your optimal aerobic training zone and you want to add to your workout. Gardening activities throughout the year will wax and wane. Adding a few sit-ups, pull-ups, and step-ups a couple of dozen times will help provide a balanced *Get Fit through Gardening* workout.

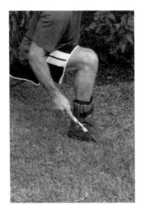

SINCE *Get Fit through Gardening* emphasizes the legs, wearing leg weights may not be necessary. However, on light aerobic days, it will help tone the legs more and burn more calories. Again, as your gardening activities wind down, and your garden workouts are shorter and less intense, adding leg weights and even light arm weights is yet another creative way to increase the health benefits of gardening.

To build strength and size in your muscles, you should only be able to perform an exercise for 3 sets of 10 to 12 repetitions. Remember to rest for 30 seconds between each set, allowing your muscles time to recover and prepare for the next set.

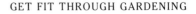

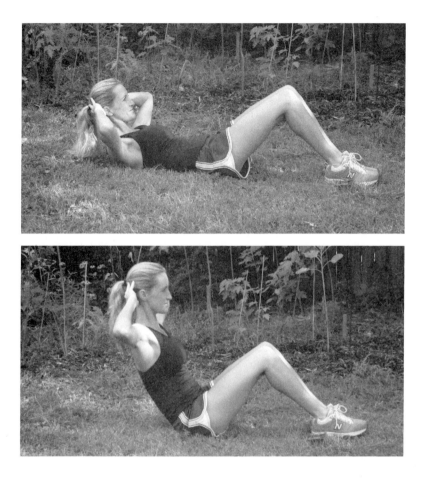

Lay on the ground with your hands behind your head, your feet flat on the ground, and your knees at a 90-degree angle. Now, move up until your back is completely off of the ground, making sure not to use your feet or your hands to push off. Be aware of any outside momentum not coming from your abs. Lower yourself back to the ground.

91

Bicycles

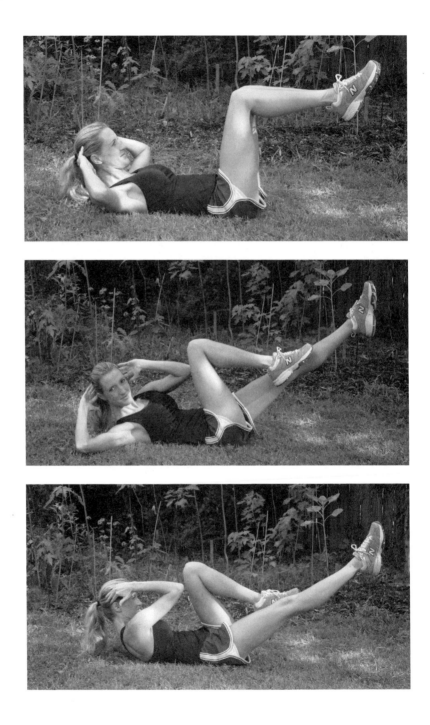

Lay on the ground with your hands behind your head and your feet in the air so that your calves are parallel to the ground. Crunch across your body while simultaneously scissoring your legs out, bringing your right elbow to touch your left knee. At this point your right leg should be completely extended. Now, crunch backwards and switch sides.

Push-Ups

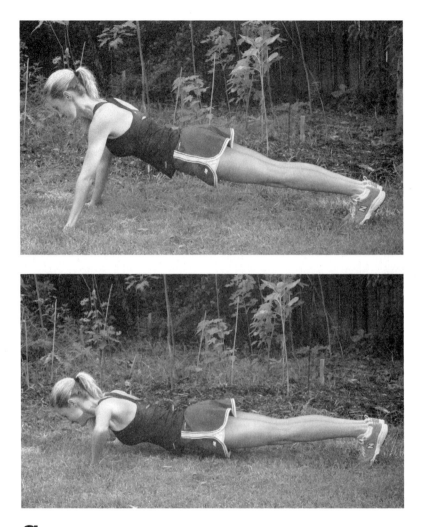

Get into the plank position, your hands at shoulder width. Carefully lower yourself to the ground so that your head is 2 to 3 inches from the ground. Raise yourself and repeat. This classic exercise works the pectorals and the triceps.

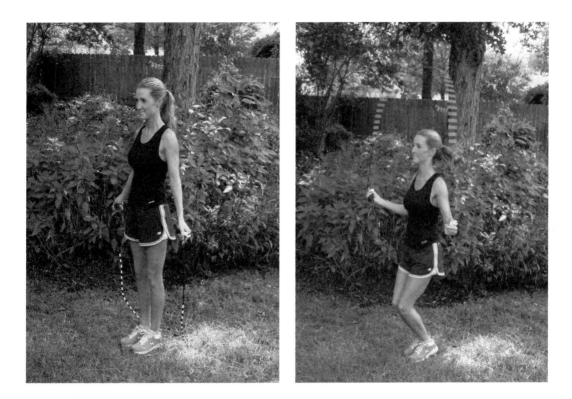

An excellent way to rev yourself up and prepare for the work-out ahead is to use a cardio tool like a jump rope. Vigorously jump rope for 5 to 10 minutes. Get that blood pumping!

Step-Up Box

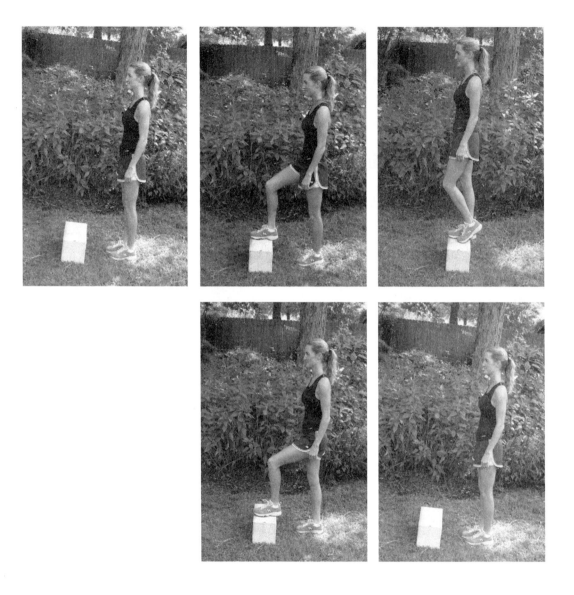

Set up a wooden box, cinder block, or a plastic step in your backyard between garden beds. There's no construction involved and it's another reminder that you are working out as you garden. Every time you pass the box, step up 20 times, alternating legs each time.

Calf Raises

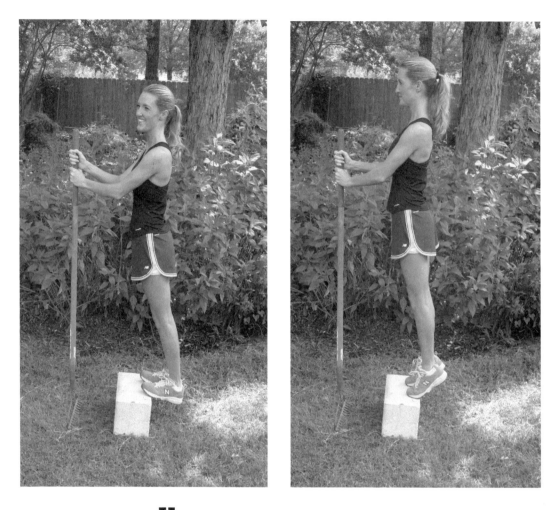

Use your box as a tool to increase the workout of your calf muscles. You will need a pole or long-handled tool in range to keep you steady for this workout. Stand on the edge of your box so that your heels are hanging off and only the balls of your feet are on the box. Slowly lower your heels down an inch or two, being careful not to go too low, and raise yourself. Repeat 10 to 12 times.

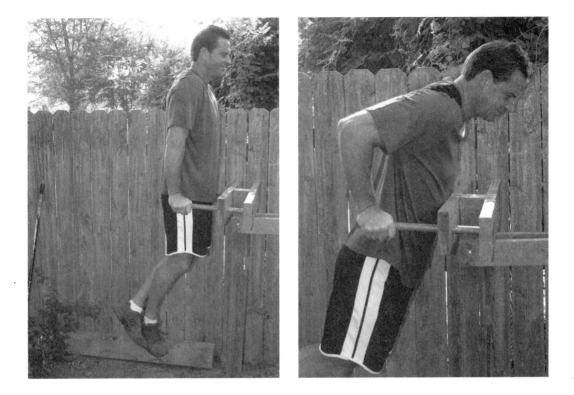

A dip bar is a relatively easy structure to create out of metal pipe and treated wood. I use iron plumbing pipe and 2 × 6 wood mounted on a 4 × 4 post. Be sure to use a distance between the two bars that is comfortable for you. Dips are a great exercise for your pectoral muscles and triceps. If you have difficulty doing them, set up a box underneath you so you can support your weight. The number of dips you can perform is based on your strength/weight ration. Dips are another great test of overall fitness compared to your weight.

Grasp the bars firmly, and raise yourself up so that your elbows are not quite locked. Raise your feet off of the ground so your knees make a 90-degree angle. Slowly lower yourself to the ground until your elbows make a 90-degree angle. Raise yourself back to the starting position and repeat 10 to 15 times.

Chin-Up/Pull-Up Bar

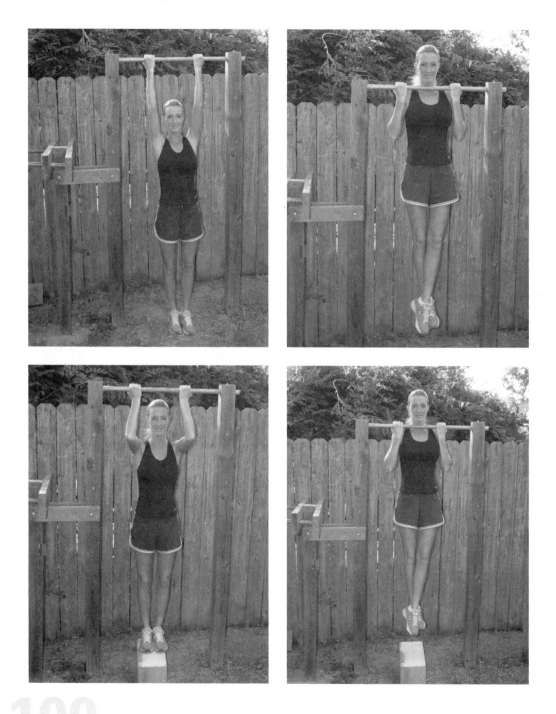

If you're able to do even a few chin-ups or pull-ups, I would highly recommend setting up a bar in your back yard. It's a simple project and a great exercise for the latissimus dorsi, biceps and forearms. Since your ability to perform chin-ups and pull-ups is based on your strength and weight, it's a great gauge of your overall fitness. If you're unable to do at least one, set up a box or a post underneath you in front of the bar or recruit a spotter to help.

Place your feet on the box and use your legs to assist with the chin-up or pull-up until your arms are stronger or your weight is low enough to perform them unassisted. Chin-ups and pull-ups can also be performed with a spotter; place your foot in the spotter's hands, and push off as necessary to complete the movements.

A chin-up is performed with your palms facing toward you. A pull-up is performed with your palms facing away from you. Otherwise the movement is the same. Generally, you can do more chin-ups than pull-ups.

Jugs of Water

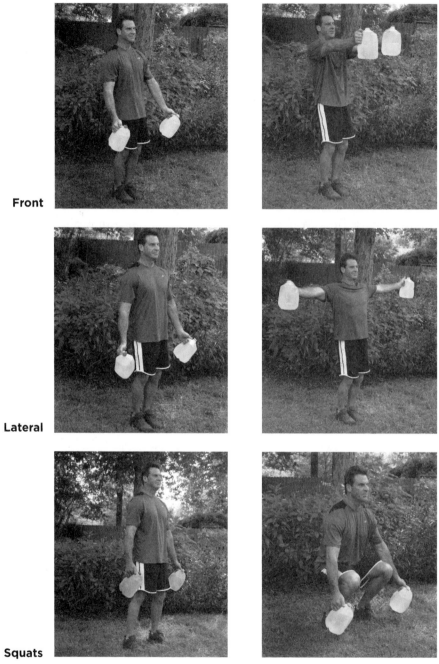

Front

Lateral

Squats

A quick way to add a strength-training component to your gardening is using this quick, full-body workout. Simply fill milk jugs full of water and keep them near your garden beds. When you're ready, slowly raise them from waist level out to the sides to shoulder level. Lower them. Slowly raise them out to your front at shoulder level. Lower them, and continue down to a squat. Return to the starting position. Perform this motion 10 times.

If it's too difficult, pour out some of the water in the jugs. You should do 3 sets of 10 repetitions of each exercise.

Attach Exercise Bands to Your Chin-Up Bar

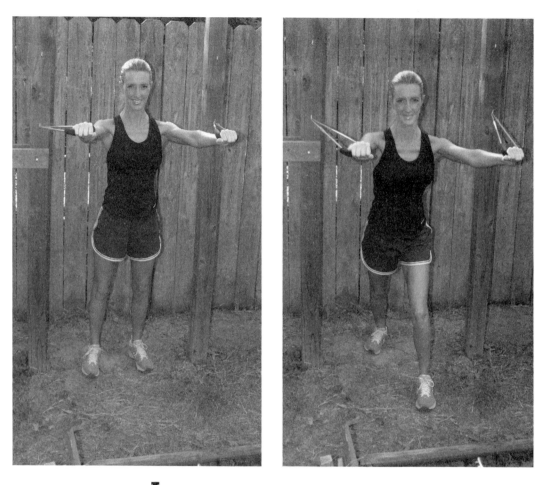

Install eye-hooks to the pull-up bar posts at different heights and use rubber exercise bands to add more resistance training to your *Get Fit through Gardening* workout. For less than 50 dollars you can create a workout very similar to expensive weight machines. Simply stand between the bars with your arms out before you grasping the bands, and lunge forward. It's your very own chest press machine!

I often use multiple bands set on eye-hooks 12 to 24 inches apart. I have 8 bands in 2 different lengths. The eye-hooks can

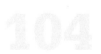

also be set up in your garage or inside a door frame. With multiple bands on eye-hooks at different heights, the number of exercises you can do is virtually endless.

Creative Outdoor Exercises

Be creative. As gardening activities decline in mid-summer, add exercises so you always reach your target aerobic zone (see p. 118). Do push-ups in between planting flowers. Skip rope for 5 minutes. Hang a rope on a tree and climb it. Setup a mini-trampoline in your backyard to add flexibility and jumping exercises with less impact on your joints and tendons. Add a commercial jungle gym for the children. Encourage them to combine the jungle gym with their gardening exercises. Set up an obstacle course using old tires. Hang an old tire from a tree, and practice throwing a football through it. Set up a soccer goal, and kick goals between weeding beds. Ideas for exercising in your garden are limited only by your imagination.

Focus On Your Breathing

EXHALE during the exertion phase and inhale during the relaxation stage. This means for most motions, you'll be exhaling during the pull phase. If you are digging a hole, inhale as you push down on the shovel and exhale as you lift the dirt and move it.

Quantifying Gardening Exercises

6

THIS IS A critical, but often overlooked component of any fitness program. To truly make the transition from traditional gardening to *Get Fit through Gardening*, you must measure, count, and quantify your gardening activity. This will greatly enhance the benefits and provide weekly feedback about your workouts' effectiveness.

Your first step should be to start a journal. If your goal is to lose weight, write down what you eat every day and record all your gardening and cross-training exercises. Be specific. Record your weight and body-fat ratio at the beginning of every week. Alternate between aerobic and resistance training sessions. Be consistent. The simple activity of journaling every day will reinforce the exercise techniques and concepts in this book.

It's important to know what your body is actually doing. For example, I walked on a treadmill at 4.5 miles per hour for years. It wasn't until I purchased a heart-rate monitor that I discovered I never achieved my optimal heart rate (at that time it was 139 beats per minute). My heart rate was under 120 bpm. For years I thought I was exercising aerobically, but I wasn't.

Counting and quantifying your activities will take concentration and might at first detract from your enjoyment of gardening. After time, adherence to repetitions, sets, and your stance will become automatic and your enjoyment of the gardening experience will *increase*.

Think Repetitions and Sets

THIS concept is borrowed from weight training. While raking and digging a hole is not exactly the same as doing a bench press, the concepts are similar. Group raking and cultivating motions first into repetitions and then sets. For example, rake ten to fifteen sweeps briskly. That's one set of fifteen repetitions. Break by doing something else for a minute, then continue raking. Each group of repetitions is called a set. You should do at least three sets. Adapt this type of thinking for the more difficult activities such as picking up bags of soil, digging, raking, or turning a compost pile. While counting will take thought and effort at first, with consistent practice, you won't even be aware of it.

WEAR A HEART-RATE MONITOR

Check and document your heart rate often during different gardening activities at different tempos. As an alternative you can take your pulse for ten seconds and multiply by six to measure your heart rate.

Know Your Optimal Aerobic Training Zone

Some also call this the "fat-burning" zone (see p. 118). Whether you garden for thirty minutes or four hours, make it a goal to reach this zone for at least twenty minutes.

Wear a Pedometer

Wear a pedometer and walk a mile before or after gardening. Also measure how many steps you take during a typical one-hour *Get Fit through Gardening* session.

> ### Always Leave Something to Do Tomorrow
>
> DON'T finish all your garden activities. Always leave a garden bed unfinished for tomorrow. If you have garden beds or raised beds, work them one at a time and always have one available for exercise.

Use Cues to Remind You to Change Your Position or Stance Often

Cues can take many forms. They can be visual, by time or sound:

1. Use a stopwatch or a watch with an alarm on it and measure how long you do an activity. Change your activity or stance every ten to fifteen minutes.

2. Use a three-minute egg-timer and alternate your raking or weeding positions every three minutes. Even if you change from a Handy Weeder to a Wrist Saver cultivator, this will balance the muscles used and reduce muscle strain.

3. Spray fluorescent paint on markers throughout the garden. When you see a new fluorescent marker, change your stance or stretch.

4. If you are listening to music as you garden, change stance or if you're kneeling, stand up every time a song changes.

5. Establish specific beds and change technique or tool used on each bed.

6. Create index cards with specific tasks listed on them. Randomly select six cards and perform each activity for five to ten minutes.

7. Use a pedometer and alternate your position every 200 steps.

Quantify Your Workout

RECORD, journal, or count what you do. Simply keeping a journal of what you eat and your workout, counting out repetitions, or wearing a heart-monitor while gardening will increase the fitness benefits.

Get Fit through Gardening Exercise Programs

7

WHAT FOLLOWS ARE sample *Get Fit through Gardening* workout programs, organized by duration and whether any additional structures are used. Remember, this is a total body workout program, and it will be necessary to "swap in" some non-gardening exercises to get the full experience.

This is a circuit training workout. Think of the different garden tools and activities as stations. Your goal is to move quickly from station to station. Planning, writing down your daily and weekly and long-term objectives, and journaling are all critical to the success of your *Get Fit through Gardening* workout. Obviously, these programs are only guidelines and whether you want to Lunge and Weed for eight minutes or twelve minutes or pick flowers for four minutes or twenty minutes will ultimately be your decision.

It's difficult to garden for only thirty minutes. But that's a good thing. While many other exercises like walking or stair-stepping are easily performed in one thirty-minute workout, *Get Fit through Gardening* is best when workouts are long enough to burn fat, but not too long as to be uncomfortable. For most gardeners, that's an hour or longer.

Vary your workout often. Once every three months, turn the compost pile. Every two or three weeks you might want to double-dig a bed. Incorporate mowing your lawn into your workout in creative ways as an aerobic warm-up or cool-down. During the spring, cleanup activities will dominate your time. In the fall and the winter, raking leaves in thirty-minute sessions will be your primary activity.

The use of structures offers many interesting variations. If most of your garden tasks are accomplished quickly you can enhance your workout by performing sit-ups, chin-ups, and step-ups.

I suggest following these programs strictly at least a few times at first, with the goal of making them an automatic, effortless activity. Rarely do I count the minutes as I perform these activities. But I instinctively stretch, change activities, and alternate stances often.

	MONDAY	WEDNESDAY	FRIDAY	SATURDAY	SUNDAY
Weeks 1-2	20 minutes Focus: Light stretching	20 minutes Focus: Flexibility and endurance test	20 minutes Focus: Light stretching	20 minutes Focus: Flexibility and endurance test	Day off
Weeks 3-4	30 minutes Medium intensity gardening	30 minutes Medium intensity gardening	20 minutes Focus: Light stretching	Day off	30 minutes Medium intensity gardening
Weeks 5-6	40 minutes Intense gardening	20 minutes Intense gardening	1 hour Light gardening	40 minutes Medium intensity gardening	Day off

Outlining and planning your workout is a critical component to the *Get Fit through Gardening* workout. Plan both your garden and your exercise. At first, *Get Fit through Gardening* will require advance planning. Instead of finishing all your yard work in one frenzied weekend, your objective now is to portion out the effort in easy increments, four to five days a week, over an extended period of time.

Have fun. Take days off. Alternate intense workouts with light workouts and short gardening sessions with longer ones. There are no rules and no score. The key is to start. Then stay with it, season after season, year and year, and decade after decade.

Muscles Used During Typical Gardening Activities

Most gardeners don't think about which muscles they use as they garden. These tables will break down individual activities to demonstrate which muscle groups are being exercised.

ARMS

EXERCISE	WRIST	FOREARMS	BICEPS	TRICEPS
Lunge and Weed	YES	YES	YES	YES
The Stance	YES	YES	(PULL IN)	(PUSH OUT)
Digging	YES	YES	YES	YES
Prunning	YES	YES		
Post -Hole Digger	YES	YES	YES	YES
Mini-Tiller Shuffle	YES	YES	YES	YES

CHEST, SHOULDERS, AND BACK

EXERCISE	TRAPEZIUS	PECTORALIS MAJOR	LATISSIMUS DORSI	DELTOIDS
Lunge and Weed	YES			YES
The Stance	YES	YES	YES	
Digging	YES	YES	YES	YES
Post-Hole Digger	YES	YES	YES	YES
Mini-Tiller Shuffle	YES	YES	YES	YES

116

Abdominals and Lower Body

EXERCISE	EXTERNAL	ABDOMINALS	QUADRICEPS	ANKLE	GLUTEUS
Lunge and Weed	YES	YES	YES	YES	YES
The Stance	YES	YES	YES	YES	YES
Digging	YES	YES	YES	YES	YES
Post-Hole Digger	YES	YES	YES	YES	YES
Mini-Tiller Shuffle	YES	YES	YES	YES	YES

Sample Workout Program: 20-Minute Workouts

For this first program, you'll spend most of your time limbering up and preparing your body for the more strenuous gardening exercises in the weeks to come. Think of the different garden tools and activities as stations and keep an eye on the clock. Your goal is to move quickly from station to station. You should change activities and alternate stances every few minutes.

Know Your Optimal Aerobic Training Zone

SOME also call this the "fat-burning" zone. Below is one way to calculate your target heart rate: Subtract your age from 220 and your aerobic training zone is between 70 and 80%.

Minus Your Age = Maximum Heart Rate			70%	80%
220	18	202	141	162
220	25	195	137	156
220	40	180	126	144
220	50	170	119	136
220	55	165	116	132
220	65	155	109	124
220	70	150	105	120
220	75	145	102	116

Wear a heart-rate monitor and record how long it takes to reach your optimal aerobic training zone as you perform the Lunge and Weed, or use the Stance. You may need to adjust your raking or digging cadence to maintain your heart rate in the zone. Some activities, like using a manual lawn aerator, won't ever achieve a true "aerobic zone" but others, like digging a hole, most certainly will.

118

	SESSION 1	SESSION 2	SESSION 3	SESSION 4
WARM UP				
Jump Rope (p.95)	2		2	
Pruning (p. 85)		2		
Stretching (p.37-59)	5	5	5	5
LIGHT ACTIVITIES				
Picking Up Objects (p.84)			2	
Full Resting Squat and Weed (p.77)	2			
Lawn Aerator (p.82)	2			
MEDIUM ACTIVITIES				
Lawnmower In and Out (p.80)		5		
Lunge and Weed (p. 70-73)	2		4	2
The Stance (p.66)	4	5		
Digging (p.82)			2	5
Post-Hole Digger (p.85)				5
Mini-Tiller Shuffle (p.29)			2	
STRENGTH-TRAINING				
Chin-Up/Pull-Up (p.100)				
Chest Dip (p.99)				
Sit-ups (p.91)				
Bicycles (p.92)				
Push-Ups (p.94)				
Step-Up Box (p.96)				
Jugs of Water (p.102)				
Exercise Bands on Chin-Up Bar (p. 104)				
COOL-DOWN				
Stretching (p.37-59)				
Sit and weed	3		3	
Harvest		3		3
TOTAL MINUTES:	**20**	**20**	**20**	**20**

SAMPLE 20-MINUTE WORKOUT PROGRAM

GET FIT THROUGH GARDENING EXERCISE PROGRAMS

Sample Workout Program: 30-Minute Workouts

This second program will get you into the garden and introduce you to the concept of the Lunge and Weed and the Stance. Intersperse the strength-training exercises between your traditional gardening. You do not need to perform all five minutes of gardening consecutively, but the two minutes of each individual strength training exercise should be performed all at once.

Think of the different garden tools and activities as stations and keep an eye on the clock. Your goal is to move quickly from station to station. You should change activities and alternate stances every few minutes.

Alternate Between Standing and Kneeling Weeding Positions

ALTERNATE often between positions and stances. Vary your movements, activity, and stance every five, ten, or fifteen minutes. An intense, one-hour *Get Fit through Gardening* session, where you alternate your stance and movement every three to four minutes, would be no different than a typical aerobics class—with the added benefit of the fun and beauty of growing something yourself. Remember, look funny; be healthy.

	SESSION 1	SESSION 2	SESSION 3	SESSION 4
WARM UP				
Jump Rope (p.95)	2			
Pruning (p. 85)				
Stretching (p.37-59)	5	5	6	5
LIGHT ACTIVITIES				
Picking Up Objects (p.84)		2		
Full Resting Squat and Weed (p.77)			3	5
Lawn Aerator (p.82)	5		2	
MEDIUM ACTIVITIES				
Lawnmower In and Out (p.80				
Lunge and Weed (p. 70-73)	5		2	5
The Stance (p.66)	5		2	
Digging (p.82)		5		
Post-Hole Digger (p.85)				5
Mini-Tiller Shuffle (p.29)		5		
STRENGTH-TRAINING				
Chin-Up/Pull-Up (p.100)	2			2
Chest Dip (p.99)		2		
Sit-up (p.91	2			2
Bicycles (p.92)		2		
Push-Ups (p.94)	2			
Step-Up Box (p.96)		2		3
Jugs of Water (p.102)		2	2	2
Exercise Bands on Chin-Up Bar (p. 104)		2		
COOL-DOWN				
Stretching (p.37-59)				
Sit and weed	1	3		
Harvest	1		3	1
TOTAL MINUTES:	**30**	**30**	**20**	**30**

SAMPLE 30-MINUTE WORKOUT PROGRAM

Sample Workout Program: 40- to 60- Minute Workouts

To increase variety, you can intersperse the strength training exercises between your traditional gardening. Remember, the minutes assigned for each individual strength-training exercise should be performed without resting.

Think of the different garden tools and activities as stations and keep an eye on the clock. Your goal is to move quickly from station to station. You should change activities and alternate stances every few minutes.

Range of Motion

INCREASE your "Range of Motion" when raking or hand-weeding by increasing the sweep or arc, from starting position to ending position, as wide as possible. Exaggerate your motion. At first, this will take some conscious effort and practice but it will increase both caloric expenditures and the muscles used. For those familiar with a standing barbell or dumbbell curl, it's the difference between curling using a very short motion versus always going down to your waist with a fully outstretched arm. The wider Range of Motion provides a superior workout.

	SESSION 1	SESSION 2	SESSION 3	SESSION 4
WARM UP				
Jump Rope (p.95)	5		5	5
Pruning (p. 85)		5	5	
Stretching (p.37-59)	5	5	5	5
LIGHT ACTIVITIES				
Picking Up Objects (p.84)			5	
Full Resting Squat and Weed (p.77)			5	5
Lawn Aerator (p.82)			5	
MEDIUM ACTIVITIES				
Lawnmower In and Out (p.80)				15
Lunge and Weed (p. 70-73)	5	5	5	
The Stance (p.66)		5	5	5
Digging (p.82)	5			
Post-Hole Digger (p.85)		5		5
Mini-Tiller Shuffle (p.29)	5		5	
STRENGTH-TRAINING				
Chin-Up/Pull-Up (p.100)		2	2	
Chest Dip (p.99)	2			2
Sit-up (p.91)		2	2	
Bicycles (p.92)	2			2
Push-Ups (p.94)			2	
Step-Up Box (p.96)	4			4
Jugs of Water (p.102)	2		2	2
Exercise Bands on Chin-Up Bar (p. 104)			2	
COOL-DOWN				
Stretching (p.37-59)		5		5
Sit and weed		5	5	
Harvest	5	1		5
TOTAL MINUTES:	**40**	**40**	**60**	**60**

SAMPLE 40- TO 60- MINUTE WORKOUT PROGRAM

Lawn Care Workout

For the lawn care workout, you'll begin by stretching and move on to a good limbering up using your trusty jump rope. You should divide your thirty minutes of pushing the lawnmower in thirds, stopping to Lunge and Weed for a minute or two around trees or sidewalks. At the end, cool down by sitting and finishing your weeding.

Alternate Between Right-Handed and Left-Handed Raking Stances

YOU only have to switch positions for a few minutes. The switch helps balance the muscles used and the monotony of a repetitious task. This is another task that with consistent use will eventually become second nature.

	SESSION 1	SESSION 2	SESSION 3	SESSION 4
WARM UP				
Jump Rope (p.95)	5	5	5	5
Pruning (p. 85)				
Stretching (p.37-59)	5	10	10	10
LIGHT ACTIVITIES				
Picking Up Objects (p.84)			5	
Full Resting Squat and Weed (p.77)				5
Lawn Aerator (p.82)				5
MEDIUM ACTIVITIES				
Lawnmower In and Out (p.80)	30	30	30	30
Lunge and Weed (p. 70-73)	5	5	10	10
The Stance (p.66)	5			5
Digging (p.82)				
Post-Hole Digger (p.85)		5		5
Mini-Tiller Shuffle (p.29)			10	
STRENGTH-TRAINING				
Chin-Up/Pull-Up (p.100)				5
Chest Dip (p.99)		5		5
Sit-up (p.91)		5		5
Bicycles (p.92)		3	3	
Push-Ups (p.94)		2	2	
Step-Up Box (p.96)				5
Jugs of Water (p.102)		5		
Exercise Bands on Chin-Up Bar (p. 104)				
COOL-DOWN				
Stretching (p.37-59)	5		10	10
Sit and weed	5		5	10
Harvest				5
TOTAL MINUTES:	**60**	**75**	**90**	**120**

LAWN CARE WORKOUT

125

Gardening for Fitness

This sample gardening week will have you gardening in earnest. Notice how you are not performing the same task every session, but are alternating and allowing your muscles to rest. Remember, the minutes assigned for each individual strength training exercise should be performed all at once.

Think of the different garden tools and activities as stations and keep an eye on the clock. Your goal is to move quickly from station to station. You should change activities and alternate stances every few minutes.

Some Muscles Are Used More Often

GARDENING exercises most of the muscles of the body, but some more than others. The ones most often used are the shoulders, the chest, and back. With *Get Fit through Gardening* we want to transfer the emphasis to the legs, buttocks, and torso.

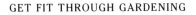

	SESSION 1	SESSION 2	SESSION 3	SESSION 4
WARM UP				
Jump Rope (p.95)	5		5	
Pruning (p. 85)		5		5
Stretching (p.37-59)	5	5	5	5
LIGHT ACTIVITIES				
Picking Up Objects (p.84)				
Full Resting Squat and Weed (p.77)	5			
Lawn Aerator (p.82)		5		
MEDIUM ACTIVITIES				
Lawnmower In and Out (p.80)				
Lunge and Weed (p. 70-73)	5	5		2
The Stance (p.66)	5		5	5
Digging (p.82)			5	
Post-Hole Digger (p.85)		5		5
Mini-Tiller Shuffle (p.29)	5		5	
STRENGTH-TRAINING				
Chin-Up/Pull-Up (p.100)		5		5
Chest Dip (p.99)	5		5	
Sit-up (p.91)		2		2
Bicycles (p.92)			2	
Push-Ups (p.94)		2		2
Step-Up Box (p.96)	2		3	
Jugs of Water (p.102)				2
Exercise Bands on Chin-Up Bar (p. 104)		2		2
COOL-DOWN				
Stretching (p.37-59)	5	5	5	5
Sit and weed	3		5	
Harvest		4		5
TOTAL MINUTES:	**45**	**45**	**45**	**45**

Create Your Own Get Fit through Gardening *Workout*

Copy this page as many times as you need to plan out your week. Eventually, you won't need this at all. For the first few weeks or months, however, it's good to have a plan to refer to.

Garden More Intensely, but for Shorter Periods of Time

ALTERNATE *Get Fit through Gardening* sessions with traditional gardening sessions. For example, use *Get Fit through Gardening* techniques to achieve your optimal aerobic zone on Mondays, Wednesdays, and Saturdays. Garden at a more leisurely pace on Tuesdays, Thursdays, and Fridays. You don't always have to go for the burn. Do what makes sense for you.

	SESSION 1	SESSION 2	SESSION 3	SESSION 4
WARM UP				
Jump Rope (p.95)				
Pruning (p. 85)				
Stretching (p.37-59)				
LIGHT ACTIVITIES				
Picking Up Objects (p.84)				
Full Resting Squat and Weed (p.77)				
Lawn Aerator (p.82)				
MEDIUM ACTIVITIES				
Lawnmower In and Out (p.80)				
Lunge and Weed (p. 70-73)				
The Stance (p.66)				
Digging (p.82)				
Post-Hole Digger (p.85)				
Mini-Tiller Shuffle (p.29)				
STRENGTH-TRAINING				
Chin-Up/Pull-Up (p.100)				
Chest Dip (p.99)				
Sit-up (p.91)				
Bicycles (p.92)				
Push-Ups (p.94)				
Step-Up Box (p.96)				
Jugs of Water (p.102)				
Exercise Bands on Chin-Up Bar (p. 104)				
COOL-DOWN				
Stretching (p.37-59)				
Sit and weed				
Harvest				
TOTAL MINUTES:				

MY GARDENING WORKOUT

	SESSION 1	SESSION 2	SESSION 3	SESSION 4
WARM UP				
Jump Rope (p.95)				
Pruning (p. 85)				
Stretching (p.37-59)				
LIGHT ACTIVITIES				
Picking Up Objects (p.84)				
Full Resting Squat and Weed (p.77)				
Lawn Aerator (p.82)				
MEDIUM ACTIVITIES				
Lawnmower In and Out (p.80)				
Lunge and Weed (p. 70-73)				
The Stance (p.66)				
Digging (p.82)				
Post-Hole Digger (p.85)				
Mini-Tiller Shuffle (p.29)				
STRENGTH-TRAINING				
Chin-Up/Pull-Up (p.100)				
Chest Dip (p.99)				
Sit-up (p.91)				
Bicycles (p.92)				
Push-Ups (p.94)				
Step-Up Box (p.96)				
Jugs of Water (p.102)				
Exercise Bands on Chin-Up Bar (p. 104)				
COOL-DOWN				
Stretching (p.37-59)				
Sit and weed				
Harvest				
TOTAL MINUTES:				

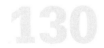

	SESSION 1	SESSION 2	SESSION 3	SESSION 4
WARM UP				
Jump Rope (p.95)				
Pruning (p. 85)				
Stretching (p.37-59)				
LIGHT ACTIVITIES				
Picking Up Objects (p.84)				
Full Resting Squat and Weed (p.77)				
Lawn Aerator (p.82)				
MEDIUM ACTIVITIES				
Lawnmower In and Out (p.80)				
Lunge and Weed (p. 70-73)				
The Stance (p.66)				
Digging (p.82)				
Post-Hole Digger (p.85)				
Mini-Tiller Shuffle (p.29)				
STRENGTH-TRAINING				
Chin-Up/Pull-Up (p.100)				
Chest Dip (p.99)				
Sit-up (p.91)				
Bicycles (p.92)				
Push-Ups (p.94)				
Step-Up Box (p.96)				
Jugs of Water (p.102)				
Exercise Bands on Chin-Up Bar (p. 104)				
COOL-DOWN				
Stretching (p.37-59)				
Sit and weed				
Harvest				
TOTAL MINUTES:				

MY GARDENING WORKOUT

	SESSION 1	SESSION 2	SESSION 3	SESSION 4
WARM UP				
Stretching (p.37-59)				
LIGHT ACTIVITIES				
MEDIUM ACTIVITIES				
STRENGTH-TRAINING				
COOL-DOWN				
Stretching (p.37-59)				
TOTAL MINUTES:				

132

	SESSION 1	SESSION 2	SESSION 3	SESSION 4
WARM UP				
Stretching (p.37-59)				
LIGHT ACTIVITIES				
MEDIUM ACTIVITIES				
STRENGTH-TRAINING				
COOL-DOWN				
Stretching (p.37-59)				
TOTAL MINUTES:				

MY CUSTOMIZED GARDENING WORKOUT

Seniors, Children, and Special Needs

8

MANY SENIOR CITIZENS (those over 65) are concerned about exercising while gardening. If you are in this number, remember that if you're already gardening—and you probably are—you are already exercising. I urge you to adopt as many of the stances and stretches in this program as possible. While you might not gain as much as someone who embraces the full workout, you will be protecting your back, knees, and muscles from injury and soreness.

Talk To Your Physician

Visit your doctor and explain to him that you will be exercising in the garden. You may need to show him this book. Explain the *Get Fit through Gardening* workout to him. Have your physician evaluate your level of fitness, check for any heart problems, and determine if you have any limitations in your back or knees. *Get Fit through Gardening* is exercise and should be taken seriously.

Garden at Your Own Pace

Next, forget the burn! Fitness experts agree there is a significant difference in the health benefits between a sedentary lifestyle and moderate exercise activity such as a half-hour walk every day. After that, health benefits from increased exercise diminish. Gardening for thirty minutes to an hour, at a steady but unhurried pace, will provide an adequate amount of physical activity for most senior citizens. In addition to the aerobic and strength-training benefits, *Get Fit through Gardening* also helps:

- decrease soreness due to repetitive motions
- balance the muscles used while gardening (alternating between standing and kneeling motions and using both a right- and left-hand raking stance)
- decrease the likelihood of injuring your back

If you're over 65, ease into *Get Fit through Gardening* by stretching for at least ten minutes several times a week. Garden for thirty minutes at least once a week, and increase to three times or more per week. Wear a heart-rate monitor while you garden and maintain 70% to 80% of your target aerobic training rate for your age. For example, if you're 75, your target range is 101.5 to 116.0 bpm.

To calculate your own target rate, just take 220, subtract your age, and multiply the result by 70% or 80% (0.70 or 0.80).

Get Fit through Gardening should never interfere with "traditional" gardening. In other words, if you garden for two hours, your goal should be to hit an aerobic training zone for at least twenty minutes. Warm-up for five minutes, stretch for ten minutes, garden aerobically (at a brisk pace elevating your heart rate) for twenty minutes, then stretch again and continue with your gardening activities (not chores) at a more relaxed pace.

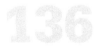

Modify These Techniques to
Meet Your Unique Physical Needs

Rather than just discounting the bending, kneeling, and squatting positions as too difficult, modify them to suit your own particular, physical needs. If kneeling or bending is too difficult, raise the garden beds to waist height with wooden or plastic planters or oak barrels. Establish garden beds that are accessible with a scooter. If you can bend but getting up is difficult, use a commercial kneeler, a walking stick, or other structure to hold onto as you lift up. If you're unable to cultivate your soil, have someone till the soil, then rake the pulverized soil at your convenience.

Ease into the raking stance gently and incrementally over a period of weeks and months. Rake for only five minutes at a time and take frequent rests. Alternate every fifteen minutes between gardening while standing, gardening while kneeling, and gardening while sitting. Whether you're 55 or 75, changing positions often and avoiding bending from your back will help you physically.

You may not be able to do chin-ups unassisted, but you may be able to do some standing on a box and using your legs underneath you as an assist. Lifting light hand weights or using a low step up box are less strenuous additions to your *Get Fit through Gardening* workout.

Garden for shorter sessions instead of long, marathon gardening sessions. Garden for shorter periods but more intensely. If you like to spend long hours in the garden, be sure to stretch thoroughly and often, follow the fundamental concepts of alternating positions often, using your legs and avoiding bending from your back.

Take normal precautions against the sun (use sun block), bugs (wear long pants, if possible), calluses (wear gloves), and eye strain (wear sunglasses). Don't wear clothes that could constrict your movements.

137

Put your personal well-being above the plants. To a lifelong gardener this might sound like heresy. Remember, with traditional gardening, the focus is on the plants. With *Get Fit through Gardening*, the focus is now on you.

Stop gardening when you're sore, tired, hot, or bored. This is not professional football and when you're injured or sore you need to rest. You want to avoid hurting or injuring your knees, back, arms, or legs.

Gardening with Bad Knees or a Bad Back

Before you begin your *Get Fit through Gardening* workout please see a specialist to determine the nature of the problem and your limitations. There is a big difference between a chronic problem that will be exacerbated by exercise and one that will be helped by steady, gradual movement.

Most of my advice for senior citizens is just common sense. Do only what is comfortable. Always stretch gently before you garden. Use long-handled tools. Change your motions and stance often. Buy a bench and sit while gardening. If you're unable to perform the Lunge and Weed as it's described, use a longer-handled tool, use a cart or stand for balance, and assume a slight bend in your knees. You may have to weed with one knee on the ground. Try to alternate knees every five to ten minutes. Never bend over from your back to pick up something. If you cannot bend down properly use a tool or a cart to pick up the object. You need to determine if stretching is possible and whether it will be helpful. Gentle stretching should be helpful but some problems, such as an anterior cruciate ligament (ACL) tear would not be helped by stretching.

Test the various new motions such as the Stance and stop if the motion hurts. Always have a support nearby when you kneel, squat or sit. Listen to your body. Know the difference between a new motion or movement and one that could potentially injure your back or knees.

Horticultural Therapy

Horticultural therapy is the application of gardening as a therapy to those who are either physically or mentally challenged. These includes those afflicted by acute illnesses such as strokes and car accidents (paraplegics, for example) and those born with a mental or physical handicap.

Conceptually, horticultural therapy is similar to *Get Fit through Gardening*. As a therapy, horticultural therapy is more concerned about helping someone with bad knees, poor eyesight, or limited mobility do something that's fun, meaningful, and provides some measure of activity, versus producing an award winning pumpkin, tomato, or rose.

Get Fit through Gardening targets the general population. The goal of *Get Fit through Gardening* is to reach everyday people who are sedentary, overweight, depressed, lonely, or bored with life.

The Horticultural Therapy Association offers a wealth of valuable information and resources for those interested in this worthwhile profession.

Gardening with Children

Gardening is a great way to wean children away from the television set and video games and help them exercise in a fun and entertaining way. Never approach gardening as a chore or punishment. Since children are conditioned to being taught by adults, learning the Lunge and Weed and the Stance won't seem so odd or unusual. Gardening is a life-long activity that is a perfect complement to television, video games, and other sedentary pursuits.

You could garden with your children, grandchildren, nieces or nephews, or even children at your church or youth group. I feel it's essential that we bring the pleasures and benefits of gardening to our youth. The *Get Fit through Gardening* workout approach can change their perceptions about gardening. The key to selling gardening as exercise is to keep the sessions short, emphasize technique, and focus on improvement and small successes.

Children are naturally more flexible than adults. The Stance will be much easier for a six-year-old than an adult. Most children can squat for hours and not even be aware of it.

Make it a competition. Teach them the concept of repetition and sets by showing them how to rake vigorously for three to five minutes then rest a few minutes. Combine raking and digging with a challenge to perform ten pull-ups by the end of the

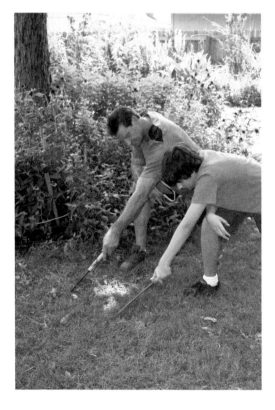

summer. Have them compete against their relatives or friends. The best part is that in addition to their ever-growing muscles and increased capabilities, they'll also have the fruits of their labor—vegetables, herbs, and flowers—to show off and enjoy.

If you present *Get Fit through Gardening* as play and not work, their imagination and creativity will flourish. Children love learning and discovering things for themselves. They will return to the garden again and again when it's fun and interesting.

Children love to accomplish a task and prove they're grown up. Small successes, so much a part of the gardening experience, have a big impact on a young child's self-esteem. Always ask them to join you in the garden. Never order them. Allowing them to follow their instincts gives them the freedom to love and appreciate the garden.

140

Establish a garden bed specifically for children. Teach them how to hold tools properly. Your young children could use those short-handled tools I advised against earlier. Add a handle to the rake. Help them prepare the soil and plant their seeds. Grow plants and vegetables that are easy to grow like zinnias, marigolds, and tomatoes.

Use a positive reinforcement system such as stickers, stars, or even cash to make it interesting. The value of some gardening activities may not be immediately apparent to small children. Therefore, the more mundane activities can carry rewards like stickers or tokens. Reward their gardening activity along with making the bed, brushing their teeth, doing their homework, and going to bed on time. Over time, they will associate gardening with the things they love, which is about the best a gardening parent can hope for.

Create a garden to attract butterflies, beneficial insects, toads, frogs, and birds. Shasta daisies, hollyhocks, ageratum, French marigolds, zinnia, tithonia, butterfly weed, and parsley all attract butterflies. Cooperating with nature instills an appreciation of its wonders. The backyard becomes a science exhibit and a wildlife habitat. In the balance of nature, beneficial insects, spiders, earthworms, birds, and toads all have a role in improving the soil or eating insect pests.

One day, when my children were young, we searched the broccoli plants for cabbage worms. My boy's eyes grew wide as he watched a parasitic wasp alight on a plant, bite a caterpillar in half, grab one end, and fly off. This might seem cruel, but it was an important lesson that no book, no television show, and no teacher could have taught better. One afternoon, my three-year-old daughter dug a hole for new tomato plants and found two white grubs in the dirt. She called them "worms" and asked me what they were doing there. I told her they lived in the dirt and would grow up to be beetles someday. My boy named one "Squirmy." They played with the two grubs for a few minutes, and he asked, "Can I squash them with my shovel?" I told him it was his choice: put them back in the dirt where they would live or squash and kill them. He thought for just a second and put them back in the dirt. I was proud of him. At the age of six, he had already gained an appreciation for life, even that of a lowly grub.

Ask children to identify the plants and vegetables they grow. Draw up flash cards with pictures of the vegetable, plant and seed on the front, and relevant growing information on the back. Work with them each year until they can identify a plant during all stages in its life cycle. Another interesting challenge is matching the seeds with the plants they grow. Always include the children when harvesting vegetables. I'll always remember picking strawberries with my children. They greeted me every day for several weeks with a request to pick the red, ripe strawberries—most were eaten before we entered the house.

Every day, the children can pick flowers for the dinner table or take them to school. They can use dried flowers for flower arrangements and crafts. Teach them to use repetitions and sets and use their legs while digging and planting. They'll learn how the effort expended in the garden provides fresh food and keeps them fit. As they grow older, they'll enjoy the garden as part of their healthy lifestyle. They can use the *Get Fit through Gardening* program with structures to prepare for team sports such as football, baseball, and soccer. Exercising in the garden can be both an alternative and complement to competitive team sports.

Succeeding at growing plants at a very young age will improve your child's self-esteem, pride, and a yearning for more. A seed planted by a small child will grow the same as one planted by a Master Gardener. The plant doesn't know or care.

The garden is an educational paradise. Children can learn about botany, agronomy, entomology, biology, chemistry, and a host of other subjects. Encouraging your children through this process and allowing their natural curiosity to flourish will open doors to many possible career opportunities. Young children have a natural curiosity about the world around them. With a little imagination and patience we can bring this exciting world of gardening and fitness to them.

Get Fit through Gardening
Activities You Can Do Today!

- 🌷 Test your soil.

- 🌷 Start a gardening/ fitness journal.

- 🌷 Join a garden club.

- 🌷 Make your garden smaller.

- 🌷 Build a compost bin.

- 🌷 Plant a fruit tree or berry bush.

- 🌷 Start a *Get Fit through Gardening* club.

- 🌷 Buy some seeds and plant them.

- 🌷 Learn to propagate plants from seeds.

- 🌷 Compost your grass clippings and leaves.

- 🌷 Prepare a five-year gardening/fitness plan.

- 🌷 Use a push mower (if your yard is small enough).

- 🌷 Learn some whole food, low-fat cooking techniques.

- 🌷 Alternate your weeding position between six positions.

- 🌷 Set up garden beds in your garden to double dig every three months.

- 🌷 Reduce or eliminate your use of chemical pesticides or herbicides.

- 🌷 Buy and use a heart-rate monitor while you garden.

- 🌷 Wear arm and leg weights while gardening for short periods of time.

- 🌷 Stretch every day whether you garden or not.

- 🌷 Record an audio tape of your ideal garden and ideal you and listen to it every day.

- 🌷 Involve a child, friend or neighbor in your *Get Fit through Gardening* lifestyle.

144

❦ Switch your stance from right to left every five minutes while raking or hoeing.

❦ Build a chin-up bar, dip bar, step-up box or other exercise structure in your yard.

❦ Warm up, stretch, elevate your heart rate and cool down while gardening.

❦ Begin a *Get Fit through Gardening* cross-training activity (walking, martial arts, yoga, or swimming).

Conclusion

IF YOU MADE it this far, then I hope that you are a new *Get Fit through Gardening* convert, ready to celebrate your fitness and wellness over the long term and by doing something that you love. How much or how little of the program you adopt is completely up to you.

While it might be challenging to change something you may have been doing all your life, and use techniques that may be unfamiliar to you, the health benefits (reducing back and muscle pain, weight loss, muscle building) are endless. Take the time, patience, and effort to learn this program, and consider someday teaching it to others, whether it's your son or daughter or a neighbor. With all the weight-loss quick fixes out there, a sound, comprehensive program like *Get Fit through Gardening* needs to be seen and heard.

While on the most basic level, this program just adds stretching, the Stance, and the Lunge and Weed to gardening, it's so much more than that. *Get Fit through Gardening* is an inexpensive, accessible, and long-term solution for the millions of people who suffer daily from obesity, diabetes, and heart disease.

Just by changing your bad gardening habits, by reading through the different suggestions and attempting the ones that make sense to you, you'll be on the route to fitness. Don't try to do everything at once. Regardless of your age, you should begin your new stretching regimen today. And remember, always garden safely.

Good luck!

—Jeff Restuccio

The Get Fit through Gardening Principles

1. This is not how your father or grandfather gardened.

2. *Get Fit through Gardening* is not work—it's exercise.

3. Never use the term "work in the garden" or "garden chores" again.

4. The focus is now on you, not the plants.

5. You garden to exercise and exercise to garden.

6. Measure success in seasons, years, and decades.

7. Adopt cross-training activities for the off-season and inclement weather.

8. Use any diet program that works for you.

9. Always follow the aerobic model.

10. Stretch before and after every *Get Fit through Gardening* workout.

11. Ease into stretching and new gardening motions gradually.

12. Make your garden smaller, not larger.

13. Garden for shorter, more intense periods.

14. Always leave something to do tomorrow.

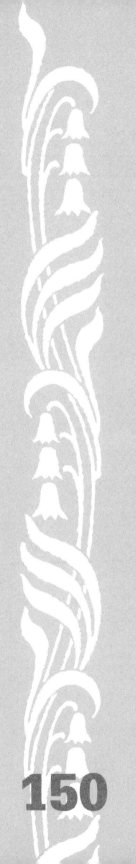

15. Always strive for a pulling/pushing motion.

16. Increase your range of motion.

17. Use reaction force (with a hand tool in both hands, pull one tool in as you push out the other.)

18. Alternate between six different weeding positions every ten minutes.

19. Alternate garden activities every ten minutes.

20. Alternate your standing stance from right- to left-handed.

21. Always, always, always use your legs and not your back.

22. Use large muscles whenever possible.

23. Never, never, never bend from your back.

24. Consistency is key.

25. Learn the Stance and this new raking motion.

26. Your knee should always be over your foot when raking.

27. Learn the Lunge and Weed.

28. Aim for your maximum aerobic training zone (for at least 20 minutes).

29. Always strive to use good exercise technique.

30. Exhale during the exertion phase while gardening.

31. Think in terms of repetitions and sets.

32. Quantify "gardening motions."

33. Wear a heart-rate monitor to develop an aerobic baseline.

34. Keep your tools razor sharp.

35. Use ergonomic tools.

36. Use long-handled tools.

37. Throw away poorly designed tools.

38. Add structures for strength training.

39. Promote National Gardening Exercise Day.

40. *The whole is more than the sum of its parts.*

Resources
and Additional
Information

Web Sites for Gardening and Fitness

www.getfitthroughgardening.com
Visit my website to learn more about the *Get Fit through
Gardening* principles and share tips on tools and exercises with
other gardeners.

www.gardenfitness.com
  The only other website I know of with tips on
  how to combine gardening with fitness.

Tools

A. M. Leonard, Inc.
www.amleo.com
www.amleo.com/index/contactus.html
PO BOX 816, Piqua, OH 45356
  Sells Forged Handy Weeder, kneelers, knee pads.

AMES TRUE TEMPER
www.ames.com
800-833-3068
465 Railroad Avenue, Camp Hill, PA 17001
Sells Mattocks, Bush Hooks. Ames True Temper "Beet Hoes" include scuffle hoe, bent shank scuffle hoe, Action Hoe. Repair handles. Replace your short handles with 60-inch handles.

CLEAN AIR GARDENING
www.cleanairgardening.com/
2266 Monitor Street, Dallas, TX 75207
214-819-9500

GARDEN HARDWARE CO.
www.gardenhardware.com
915 Folly Rd, PMB #66, Charleston, SC 29412
888-476-4426
Sells Diamond Weeding hoe, AG Weeding Push Hoe with 60-inch handle. Ho-Mi Korean Long Plow with angled blade and 57-inch handle.

GARDENERS SUPPLY CO.
www.gardeners.com
128 Intervale Road, Burlington, VT 05401
800-955-3370
Carries a wide variety of garden tools, kneelers, Cape Cod Weeder.

GARDENING WITH EASE
www.gardeningwithease.com/gwe_fistgrip2.html
P.O. Box 302, Newbury, NH 03255
800-966-5119
Sells ergonomic tools, add-on grips, Circle Hoe.

HEART HOE
www.hearthoe.com/
1999 Buford St., Alva, FL 33920
800-728-2306

Sells a unique heart-shaped hoe, with an extendable handle that you operate with a pulling motion.

MANTIS
www.mantis.com/home.asp
1028 Street Road, Southampton, PA 18966
800-366-6268

The Mantis tiller is used for the mini-tiller shuffle.

MERRIFIELD GARDEN CENTER
www.merrifieldgardencenter.com/index.php
P.O. Box 848, Merrifield, VA 22116
703-560-6222

Sells WristSaver Claw Tools by Vertex/Garden Brands and the Natural Radius Grip(TM). Discover garden hand tools.

PETA (UK) LTD
www.peta-uk.com
Marks Hall, Margaret Roding, Dunmow, Essex CM6 1QT

Designers, manufacturers and suppliers of ergonomic tools, aids and assistive devices for people suffering from arthritis or reduced grip strength. Peta UK sells ergonomic tools with wrist cuffs and unique hand-grips.

RADIUS GARDEN, LLC
www.radiusgarden.com
P.O. Box 2506, Ann Arbor, MI 48106
734-222-8044

Also sells the Natural Radius Grip.

V & B Manufacturing
www.vbmfg.com
P.O. Box 268, Walnut Ridge, AR, 72476
800-443-1987
Sells hand mattock.

More Information on Stretching

Chabut, LaReine, and Lewis, Madeleine. *Stretching For Dummies*. NY: For Dummies, 2007.

Knopf, Dr. Karl. *Stretching for 50+*. NY: Ulysses Press, 2005.

Walker, Brad. *Anatomy of Stretching*. NY: North Atlantic Books, 2007.

More Information on Organic Gardening

Organic Gardening Magazine
www.organicgardening.com
33 East Minor St, Emmaus PA 18098-0099
610-967-5171

Bartholomew, Mel. *Square Foot Gardening*. Emmaus PA: Rodale Press, 1981.

Creasy, Rosalind. *The Complete book of Edible Landscaping*. San Francisco CA: Sierra Club, 1982.

Hunt, Marjorie B. and Brenda Bortz. *High-Yield Gardening*, Emmaus PA: Rodale Press, 1986.

Rodale, J. I. *Encyclopedia of Organic Gardening*. Emmaus PA: Rodale, 1978.